Pg. 66 - 5 step
Visualization - weight
LOSS

Pg. 84 & 85
5-tips) committed to Losing

# Think Yourself Thin

Green Smoothies for Life

ALSO BY JJ SMITH

*Lose Weight Without Dieting or Working Out*

*10-Day Green Smoothie Cleanse*

*6 Ways to Lose Belly Fat Without Exercise*

*Green Smoothies for Life*

# Think Yourself Thin

A 30-Day Guide to
Permanent Weight Loss

JJ Smith

**ATRIA** PAPERBACK

NEW YORK   LONDON   TORONTO   SYDNEY   NEW DELHI

**ATRIA**
PAPERBACK

An Imprint of Simon & Schuster, Inc.
1230 Avenue of the Americas
New York, NY 10020

First Atria Paperback edition September 2018

**ATRIA** PAPERBACK and colophon are trademarks of Simon & Schuster, Inc.

For information about special discounts for bulk purchases, please contact Simon & Schuster Special Sales at 1-866-506-1949 or business@simonandschuster.com.

The Simon & Schuster Speakers Bureau can bring authors to your live event. For more information or to book an event, contact the Simon & Schuster Speakers Bureau at 1-866-248-3049 or visit our website at www.simonspeakers.com.

Interior design by Dana Sloan

Manufactured in the United States of America

10 9 8 7 6 5 4 3 2 1

Library of Congress Cataloging-in-Publication Data
Names: Smith, J. J. (Jennifer), author.
Title: Think yourself thin : a 30-day guide to permanent weight loss / JJ Smith.
Description: First 37 Ink/Atria Books trade paperback edition. | New York : 37 Ink/Atria, 2018.
Identifiers: LCCN 2018030069 (print) | LCCN 2018031496 (ebook)
Subjects: LCSH: Weight loss. | Weight loss—Psychological aspects. | BISAC: HEALTH & FITNESS / Weight Loss. | HEALTH & FITNESS / Diets. | HEALTH & FITNESS / Healthy Living.
Classification: LCC RM222.2 (ebook) | LCC RM222.2 .S622374 2018 (print) | DDC
613.2/5—dc23
LC record available at https://lccn.loc.gov/2018030069

ISBN 978-1-5011-7713-2
ISBN 978-1-5011-7714-9 (ebook)

# Contents

# Important Note to Readers

The information contained in this book is for your education. It is not intended to diagnose, treat, or cure any medical condition or dispense medical advice. If you decide to follow the plan, you should seek the advice and counsel of a licensed health professional and then use your own judgment.

It is important to obtain proper medical advice before you make any decisions about nutrition, diet, supplements, or other health-related issues discussed in this book. Neither the author nor the publisher is qualified to provide medical, financial, or psychological advice or services. The reader should consult an appropriate healthcare professional before heeding any of the advice given in this book.

# Think Yourself Thin

# Introduction

I F YOU'RE READING this book, you've probably tried a lot of diets. You may have been successful dropping a few pounds but probably gained them back and then some. At times, it feels like no matter what you eat, your body bloats and gains fat even if you just look at food. You know that there has to be an easier way to lose weight, especially given your determination and willingness to follow numerous diets and weight-loss plans. Yet you haven't figured it out. There must be something you're missing because excess weight is an ongoing issue for you.

You're not alone. The vast majority of dieters who lose weight will gain it all back within three to five years. As a result, they become frustrated and never achieve their desired weight-loss goal. The purpose of this book is to equip dieters with the most overlooked factors in dieting: the mental strategies required for permanent weight loss. Dieters know there is more to weight loss than "eat less and exercise," and this book will provide the missing piece they need to win at weight loss once and for all.

As a weight-loss expert who has written three bestselling books and developed a weight-loss system known as DHEMM,

1

I have helped dieters lose over two million pounds in two years. In so doing, I have realized that the most important, yet most overlooked, factor for permanent weight loss is mental mastery. Dieters need the mental fortitude to stay the course and finish strong. According to market research, Americans spend over $60 billion trying to lose weight every year. However, given the rising obesity rate, there is no evidence suggesting that dieting makes people healthier or thinner. In fact, statistics show that 90 percent of people who lose weight on a diet gain it back within three to five years. If people don't overcome the mental challenge of weight loss, they will struggle with weight their entire life. This is particularly detrimental because repeated dieting causes a cascade of negative psychological consequences as well.

Few books reveal the most important factor for permanent weight loss: how to create a permanent shift in thoughts, feelings, habits, and behaviors. Most diets can bring about short-term weight loss, but if they don't address the spiritual or emotional issues tied to behavior, permanent weight loss will be an ongoing challenge. You have to get to the root cause of why you're overweight. By applying what you learn in this book, you'll have the tools you need to take control of your health and weight and experience the joy of having your dream body.

## WHY EVEN LOSE WEIGHT?

Being overweight is not a crime. It doesn't devalue who you are as a person. However, weight can affect your health and overall quality of your life. It can affect almost every area of your life, including your career and personal relationships. It can affect your ability to enjoy activities with your kids. It can affect the opportunities you get on the job. It can affect the quality of mate you are able to attract and date. If you have found the quality of your life negatively impacted by your weight, make the decision to get to a healthy weight and do it.

Don't think of losing weight as just a number on the scale. When you say you want to lose weight, what you're really saying is that you want to live a long, healthy life and enjoy your kids and grandkids. When you say you want to lose weight, you are saying you want to look in the mirror and love what you see and be proud of your body. When you say you want to lose weight, you are saying you want to live life to the fullest.

## SO, DO WE GIVE UP ON TRYING TO LOSE WEIGHT?

There are numerous diets on the market that yield different results for different people. Advocates of the green smoothie cleanse, which I developed and which focuses on fast, healthy weight loss, have lost over two million pounds. Other plans focus on less carbs, more protein, but you have to be careful with the weight-loss plan you choose as some will help you not only to lose fat, but muscle as well. However, you want to maintain muscle mass as it will increase your strength and cause you to burn more fat, even while your body is at rest.

So the first thing to do is to choose the most effective weight-loss program for you, while also focusing on the mental and behavioral changes required for long-term success.

You have to decide you're done with dieting, which only results in temporary weight loss; your goal is permanent weight loss. The problem with dieting is that it doesn't help most people transition to a healthier lifestyle. The goal for permanent success is to aim for lasting change and a healthy lifestyle. Too many people think of weight loss as being about whether to try this fad diet or that fad diet, whether to count calories, eat low to no carbs, or load on the protein. The goal in these instances is to lose weight fast. But the most important thing for permanent weight loss is *sustaining* a healthy lifestyle for life. To be successful, you have to focus on the mental strategies to achieve weight-loss success.

• • •

Too many books on weight loss focus on counting calories or eliminating one thing, carbs for example, or another. There is nothing wrong with learning about the foods we eat and the impact they have on our health and weight. However, that should not be the only focal point for those looking for long-term success. The real solution is mental mastery.

## WEIGHT LOSS REQUIRES NEW HABITS AND BEHAVIORS

With my mental mastery approach, you will have to form new habits and maintain consistency. Consistency becomes the evidence of true behavioral change. It is an approach focused not on what to eat or how much exercise to get but rather on changing daily habits that will improve both mind and body. This is a timeless solution that will help you achieve your weight-loss goals for a lifetime.

Your weight is a result of current and past habits. So, logically, a different set of habits and behaviors will create a different result. You can learn a new set of habits, which will serve as the foundation for healthy living—not to stick to a diet but to live a healthy lifestyle for a lifetime. This is not to say that you will never regain some weight—there are many lifestyle factors (like having a baby, hormonal imbalances, stress) that cause weight gain. However, you will have the foundation for modifying and creating new habits to ensure you maintain a healthy body weight. Establishing new habits will ensure consistent action over time.

Most of the diet and nutrition books on the market only focus on what to eat and what not to eat. Few books focus on why we struggle with our weight and eating habits. Most people have enough understanding of what to eat, so this book is intended to serve as the complementary piece to your diet to ensure that you can create lasting change and get to your goal weight. This book will help you transform not only your body but your mind as well. You will have an improved relationship with food. You will learn how to maintain a healthy body and have great energy through positive daily habits. Not only good nutrition but also a transformed mind will keep the body healthy and attractive.

## WHAT'S IN THIS BOOK?

The great news about this book is that it is compatible with all diet plans. This book is filled with simple strategies for achieving the success you desire and for addressing every challenge you have had with your weight in the past.

In Part 1: "Five Stages of Weight Loss," we go through the psychological stages required to lose weight and keep it off. I will take you through the five stages, from being fed up with your current weight to finally getting to your ideal weight. I will help you understand the psychological process that will help you address your eating habits, food addictions, and overall health and weight issues. These are the five stages that you should expect to go through to lose weight and keep it off once and for all. I will guide you through them, one stage at a time, so that you are mentally prepared for what's to come on this journey.

Part 2: "The Solutions: Seven Mental Strategies for Weight-Loss Success," introduces the SUCCESS System, which teaches you seven new mental strategies, habits, and approaches to permanent weight loss.

1. **SLAY RESISTANCE:** *Stop Procrastination Once and For All.* Learn how to slay resistance, the most toxic force in the world. Resistance is that lethargic or apathetic feeling of not wanting to do something you know is good for you. Resistance causes us to procrastinate or delay starting something that is good for us. You must slay resistance in order to achieve the success you desire.

2. **USE VISUALIZATION:** *Use Visualization Techniques for Weight Loss.* An effective approach to losing weight permanently is to use visualization to get your mind and body to work together to get slim. Folks have had amazing results with visualization without having to starve themselves or deprive the body in any way. Visualization is a mind-body approach that makes perma-

nent weight loss easy and sustainable. I will teach you how to allow your mind to work with your body to transform yourself from the inside out.

3. **COMMIT:** *Learn How to Commit to Losing Weight.* Are you merely interested in losing weight or are you committed to losing weight? If you're truly committed, you'll do what it takes and make the necessary sacrifices. People fail not because of lack of interest or desire but because of lack of commitment. Learn the different types of motivation and how to apply them to your journey.

4. **CONTROL EMOTIONS:** *Don't Eat Your Heart Out.* Learn the signals (such as boredom, depression, loneliness, frustration, anger) that trigger emotional eating. These are the wake-up calls that let us know we're dealing with toxic emotions that need to be processed and managed.

5. **ESTABLISH SUCCESS HABITS:** *Design Your Life for Weight-Loss Success.* You can't rely on willpower and self-control to lose weight—you have to control your environment and circumstances. Your ability to maintain self-control will depend on your environment. If your house is hectic and chaotic, or if you're stressed or in a bad mood or easily distracted, you will struggle to maintain self-control. All of these circumstances can happen each and every day, so in order to have more self-control, you will have to change your environment by establishing success habits.

6. **SUPPORT FROM OTHERS:** *Have a Support System in Place.* Studies show that those who have a support community

have more long-term success with weight loss. Learn how to create support systems and accountability partners.

7. **SUPERCHARGE YOUR SPIRITUAL LIFE:** *Tap into Your Spiritual Power to Achieve Weight-Loss Success*. Until your mind and spirit are engaged in your weight-loss efforts, excess weight will continue to be a problem for you. The ultimate problem is not your physical weight but what is happening in your mind and spirit causing you to gain weight.

Part 3: "30-Day Mental Mastery Challenge" provides thirty days of exercises supporting the strategies taught in the SUCCESS System to ensure you can create new habits and behaviors that create lasting and permanent weight loss for life.

Part 4: "Motivational Success Stories," provides over fifteen motivational success stories and pictures of how others overcame poor eating habits, health issues, low motivation, and depression to lose the weight and keep it off. If they did it, you can too!

The book also includes an appendix, "Twelve Principles for Clean and Balanced Eating." No matter what you have learned in the past, these twelve principles provide the guidance you need to eat in a manner that helps the body burn fat and lose weight. These guiding principles allow you to maximize your weight loss while following the strategies taught in this book.

I will be totally transparent with you. The SUCCESS System calls for complete honesty. You will need to be honest with yourself. In order to create change in your life, you have to admit to the mistakes and decisions that have caused you to struggle for so long. If you are really ready for a new body and a new life, then keep reading.

## CONGRATULATIONS!

I want to congratulate you for having the courage to take back control of your weight and your health. I know how much courage it takes to begin a new life and a new relationship with food. I support you and encourage you in your efforts.

I have had frustrations with unexplained weight gain. I have worked hard to lose weight only to find that each week the pounds continued to pile on. But know that everything we need to turn our dreams into a reality is within us. We are fully equipped to achieve our weight-loss goals. I hope this book will challenge you to use the God-given power within you to transform your mind, body, and spirit. There are tips and strategies that will allow you to produce measurable, long-lasting changes to achieve your health and weight-loss goals.

While this is not a typical "diet" book, by following the strategies outlined here, you will experience weight loss. More important, you will adopt a whole new perspective on weight loss. This journey will challenge you, but the pursuit of greatness and happiness rarely comes without effort. Trust that your body will reward you for your efforts, if you just stay consistent throughout this journey.

I suggest you read this book one time through for understanding, then reread it to begin your journey by applying the strategies. I provide healthy weight-loss plans that will yield results, and this book complements my weight-loss plan or any diet on the market. The key to lasting results is transforming the mind.

In addition, support will be very helpful to you on this journey. I urge you to get a copy of the book for a family member and friend so that you all can encourage each other through this life-changing transformation. Join seven hundred thousand others who get free support from me and my team on a daily basis on our Facebook page at: https://www.facebook.com/groups/Green.Smoothie.Cleanse/.

Your family, friends, and I will be here to guide you along and support you. You are not alone. We will do this together. Let your journey begin today.

Sincerely,
JJ Smith

# Part One

---

## FIVE STAGES OF WEIGHT LOSS

Weight loss is a process. In this section, we will go through the psychological stages required to both lose weight and maintain weight loss.

I will take you through the five stages, from being fed up with your current weight to finally getting to your ideal weight. I will help you understand the psychological process that is normal and expected to help you address your eating issues, food addictions, and overall health and weight issues. These are the five stages that you should expect to go through to lose weight and keep it off once and for all. I will guide you through them, one stage at a time, so that you are mentally prepared for what's to come on this journey.

Even if you only have 10 pounds to lose, the fact that you are reading this book means you realize that you need or want to lose weight. So you are in the right place. You're ready to face your weight problems, and this takes great courage. You have the power to change your weight and improve the quality of your health. Weight-loss success is within your control.

# 1

## Stage One—Fed Up

THERE ARE MANY overweight or obese people who don't think they actually have a weight problem. They have no desire or intention of changing their lifestyle. They might actually be happy in their overweight state; however, most are not. They will make excuses like "I'm too busy to lose weight" or "My husband loves me just the way I am." But the truth is that most overweight people also have or will develop health issues that jeopardize their chance of a long, prosperous life.

Many overweight people can live in fat denial for years before something causes them to realize that they are overweight and that they have to do something about it. The National Weight Control Registry began a study in 1994 to track successful weight-losers, whom they call Weight Loss Masters. Weight Loss Masters are those who have lost at least 30 pounds or more and have kept it off for a year or more. One finding was that nearly 80 percent of Weight Loss Masters began their weight-loss journey due to a triggering event. A triggering event is a situation, event, or may even be a comment that makes you think about something differently. The triggering event is what is needed to get out of fat denial and on to taking action. Fat denial for me happened when I would wear slacks and just unbutton the top button or wear stretchy leggings and big sweatshirts. This was my attempt to deny the fact of my excess weight.

To move on to the next phase, we have to come out of fat denial and realize that we need to do something differently.

## HOUSTON, WE HAVE A PROBLEM, THE TRIGGERING EVENT

Once you realize you are fat, overweight, or obese—whatever you choose to call it—there has to be a clear acknowledgment of the problem. You may not know whether you are eating the wrong foods, struggling with emotional eating, or have hormonal imbalances that are causing weight gain, but you know there is a problem. All real growth happens in life when we acknowledge that there is a problem that needs to be addressed.

Marie had a problem with her weight ever since high school. Food always comforted her, but it also became her "boo." She got comfort and companionship from food rather than from a mate. She would go on diets in which she would see food as her enemy, but ultimately she would always go back to her first love, food. In her twenties she stopped dieting, and just embraced the love she had for food. When it came to eating, it was all love, all the time. Food was her friend, her companion, her joy, her lover.

One day, Marie went to the movies alone and, as usual, brought her own food—cakes and cookies were her favorites. She saw Jennifer Aniston on the screen and thought she was so small and cute. I wish I could look like that, she thought, as she stuffed another cookie in her mouth. She didn't acknowledge that she had a problem that needed to be addressed. She didn't acknowledge that she was fat and needed to do something about it. She just wore baggy sweaters and leggings and made herself as comfortable as possible.

Then one day, she was walking through the mall and caught a glimpse of a woman in the mirror who made her think Wow, that lady is so big! She also noticed that this lady was wearing the same outfit she had put on that day. So she stopped and looked more closely. She quickly realized she was walking toward a mirror and that woman was her! That was her triggering event, the turning point that motivated her to see she was fat and to embrace the fact that she needed to lose weight. At that moment, she knew she needed to get real and do something about her weight.

I coach thousands of folks in my private weight-loss coaching group, and one benefit of it is that folks can learn from the success others are having at losing weight. As discussed above, 80% of Weight Loss Masters, those who have lost at least 30 pounds or more and have kept it off for a year or more, began their weight-loss journey due to a triggering event. The triggering event is what is needed to get out of fat denial and on to taking action.

Sometimes, when you gain a lot of weight, you really don't see it. You may feel it when your thighs rub together or your knees ache, but you can't see it in a mirror. Others often see it before you do. Be grateful if you have a relative who will let you know that you've picked up a few pounds.

Looking at recent photos and not recognizing yourself is another potential trigger. All of your beautiful curves are gone because you have become so rotund.

Once you get out of fat denial, you can face the reality of the work that is necessary to lose weight and keep it off.

## REALIZING THAT YOU HAVE A PROBLEM

So many people realize that they have been fat the majority of their life. Even when they look back at photos of themselves, they can't find a single photo where they weren't chubby or overweight.

Others gained weight after they went to college. First, there is the "freshman 15"—the 15 pounds many students gain during the freshman year of college. Most college students gain about 25 pounds total during their college years. Many assume it's due to the high-starch cafeteria foods.

Another time of significant weight gain is once a person gets married. Women, in particular, do great to keep themselves up when they're trying to get a husband, but after they get one, they let themselves go. They feel secure in the fact that they have found someone to love them for life. Also, during marriage we cook more frequently, care for others more often and, as a result, have a tendency to neglect ourselves. Consequently, the weight starts to pile on.

A married girlfriend of mine came to me one day and said she needed my help to lose weight. She had a sense of urgency, and I asked her why. She'd been carrying the extra weight for years. She said her husband had told her he wasn't physically attracted to her anymore. She said, "I first got mad, but then I realized I had a choice. I could stay overweight and risk him finding someone else, or get it together and be the woman he married!" She had chosen the latter. She did lose the weight, and today they are still happily married. So, while it may have initially hurt to have had a family member be honest with her, it was ultimately helpful.

Many women gain weight after having their first child. It is perfectly normal to gain weight in pregnancy, but many women struggle to get their body back and find it hard to lose the "baby weight." Some women who have more than one child keep gaining more and more weight with each one.

No matter what the reason is for the weight gain, there must be some acknowledgment that you are overweight before you can decide to do something about it. When you have acknowledged that you are overweight but haven't done anything about it, it can be a very painful place to be. But it's a necessary first step. As the expression goes, it's always darkest before the dawn.

Don't be afraid, go ahead and get on the scale. Write the number down. Take photos, take your measurements. Come out of denial with power and courage. For your weight is truly about to change.

## THE DECISION HAS BEEN MADE

Now that you have made the decision to lose weight, you will have enough motivation to begin this journey. Coming out of fat denial frees you up to use your mental energy to focus on losing weight and getting healthy as opposed to using it to defend being overweight. Living in truth will set you free.

All the Weight Loss Masters went through this stage too and they unanimously report that it's liberating to go from "I'm fat!" to "I'm ready to make a change!"

In my experience coaching thousands of folks on their weight-loss journey, I have seen that the reasons for losing weight generally fall into one of three categories:

1. **VANITY:** You don't like the way you look or you never attract the opposite sex. The pressure could be external, such as you get teased because of your weight. Or internal—you might look in the mirror and simply not like what you see.
2. **QUALITY OF LIFE:** You want to spend quality time with your family, especially your mate, kids, and grandkids. If you are struggling to run and play with your children, it will only get worse if you don't address it now.
3. **HEALTH:** Not only is your health failing, you have no energy to actively participate in life. The doctor may have ordered you to lose weight due to weight-related illnesses such as high blood pressure, diabetes, or high cholesterol. Your body is failing you and your back, knees, and feet hurt all the time due to excess weight.

Be careful of the "I'll start next week" syndrome. Monday is the most popular start date and the most procrastinated start date as well. How many times have you said, I'll start my new weight-loss plan next week, on Monday? This might be an excuse to overeat on the weekends and eat everything in sight for a few days. You overeat without feeling guilty, but then when Monday comes and goes and you haven't started, you end up feeling even worse. This is a set-up for failure. If you make a decision to lose weight, create a game plan today and get started today. There is nothing magical about Monday.

Now you may have already come up with some excuses as to why today is not a good day to start. Well, don't be fearful about taking action today. This book will give you the mental strategies to stay motivated throughout your weight-loss journey. You don't need to run out and buy a gym membership or buy any weight-loss pills or foods. You just need to start eating better today.

I know you may be thinking that you have tried so many diets in the past and either couldn't stick with it or gained all the weight back. You are not alone: the majority of the people who have lost weight and kept it off have tried at least five diets or more. So, that is normal and does not make you a failure. People try low-carb diets, high-protein diets, low-fat diets, all kinds of fad diets, and then still gain the weight back. So, the diet is not the answer. Diets are simply not the most effective way to lose weight permanently. Your goal should be to change your lifestyle, including proper nutrition and getting physically active, as a way to achieve your weight-loss goals. When most people think of dieting, they immediately think of eating less, which is a flawed dieting technique that allows you to lose weight in the short term but rarely allows you to keep the weight off permanently.

Remember, no more excuses. Sure, you may love food. Most people do! No one wants to give up favorite foods entirely. I know I didn't. To this day, I still love pizza, lasagna, burgers, and fries. And I still get to eat them now and then. I just can't eat them every day and maintain my weight. So don't worry about giving up anything. There is a way to include your favorite foods and still be slim and healthy.

Keep a long list of why you want to lose weight and keep it visible so you can see it every day. Refer to it to remind yourself of why you started. On challenging days, you'll need these reminders to keep going.

# 2

---

# Stage Two—The Honeymoon (Starting Strong)

---

S O YOU MADE the decision to lose weight and you're ready to take action. It took time to come out of denial to move into action, but you're finally ready to make a lifestyle change. You no longer feel hopeless. This is the stage when you start outlining a plan to take action, and you may even start making some small changes like drinking more water, getting more sleep, or going for walks.

I admire folks who want to jump right in, but learning how to help your body lose weight is one of the most important aspects of achieving your goal. During this stage, we recommend people begin researching different weight-loss programs and getting their minds ready for change. There is so much confusing and conflicting information out there, so you want to make sure to get the right information. And no worries, I'll give you the most important information on how your body metabolizes food so that you can be successful at weight loss. That's actually the easy part. The challenge is the mental motivation, which is the focus of this entire book. It's one of the most difficult phases because you are getting rid of bad habits and replacing them with good ones.

## DEALING WITH EMOTIONAL EATING

In this phase, you will lose a good bit of weight. It will be challenging because you will also be breaking food addictions, changing eating habits, and learning how not to let emotional eating take you off track. It is a time to deal not only with inner struggles but also with family and friends who do not support the lifestyle changes you are trying to make.

When you are truly making a lifestyle change, you do not want to worry about diets and specific food choices. I never tell people what to eat. I help them understand which foods help them burn fat and which foods help them store fat so they can make educated choices when they eat. It is about being aware and making better decisions one meal at a time.

In this stage, you confront the inner struggles that contributed to your weight gain. One of the biggest struggles for many is dealing with emotional eating.

When Carol felt lonely in the past, she would eat. When she was bored, she would eat. When she felt stressed, she would eat. She finally came to the realization that she was using food to deal with her emotions, to fill up the lonely places in her life. But she was unsure what to do about it.

Some people abuse food the way addicts abuse drugs or alcohol. And just like a drug addict will go through withdrawals and discomfort when they try to break the bad habit, so does a person who is dealing with food addictions. Carol had to learn to feel every emotion she was experiencing, instead of trying to eat away her feelings. Carol had to learn to just feel lonely or bored and be aware of those feelings so she could fulfill her life in healthier ways besides eating.

She began to go to the gym, take walks, participate in online support communities. She even joined a bowling league. Bowling was something she had loved when she was younger, and joining a league helped her commit to being out of the house more often, which led to more fun in her life. She later signed up for a line-dancing class because dancing made her feel alive. Now, when Carol feels bored or lonely, she gets out of the house before she resorts to eating. She has become very aware of how important it is to leave the house to make new friends and enjoy some of her favorite activities.

Carol's story illustrates how losing weight really requires a lifestyle change—a true change of habits. No more long workdays and lonely nights. Carol keeps her free time filled with hobbies, friends, and fun; food is no longer her primary comforter. Carol will tell others how being aware of her feelings helped her change her eating habits. She had to be aware of the feelings that led to emotional eating and indulgence.

Do you eat when you are sad, hurt, bored, or lonely? Emotional eating almost always leads to inappropriate eating. Without realizing it, you may be caught in a vicious cycle of "living to eat" as opposed to "eating to live." Just like a drug or alcohol addict, you have to make sure that you do not use food to escape your problems. Food should be seen for what it is: fuel for the body to give it energy and vitality.

An important way to address emotional eating is to learn the difference between emotional hunger and physical hunger. This is absolutely key. Sometimes our relationship with food is an emotional one rather than a physical one. Sometimes we eat to fill an emotional gap or some other negative emotion. But no food—be it crackers, cake, ice cream, or pie—can satisfy emotional hunger.

Emotional hunger comes on suddenly: I must eat something now. However, you rarely feel satisfied or full, and so you just keep eating and eating until the entire bag of chips or pint of ice cream is gone. If the hunger comes on after an argument or a negative emotion, then it is emotional hunger. You need to learn to deal with the emotions head-on.

Physical hunger comes about gradually about every three to four hours. Watch the clock. If you ate a meal and were full one hour ago and then feel a sudden need to eat something, it is probably emotional hunger.

Dealing with your emotional issues will help you improve your relationship with food. To deal with your emotions, you must come to understand that the bad things that have happened in your life have probably been floating around in your mind for years, and because you try to suppress these feelings—as most of us do—they have never been properly processed.

When we dwell on the sad events of our lives, they get etched in our minds, stuck in our bodies, weighing us down emotionally. We must process these experiences and let them go. If we do not, the negative emotions become toxic to our emotional and physical body. Sad or painful experiences are meant to teach us lessons we needed to learn so that we can grow and mature as a person. They are not meant to linger for years and years.

We will discuss more about emotional hunger later in this book.

## DEALING WITH BAD HABITS

Many of us have daily routines: habits for how we get dressed, prepare breakfast, get ready for work, and prepare dinner each day. A bad habit is one that does not help us achieve our goals. A good habit makes us more productive and effective in life.

The same is true for eating habits. Good eating habits help us lose weight consistently and bad eating habits work against our efforts. If you are eating the same things, or similar things, every day and you are not losing weight, consider changing your eating habits. If what you eat is keeping you slim and healthy, then you have good eating habits.

So how do you go about changing bad habits? First, awareness is key. Think about how many things you do without even thinking about it. Some habits are at the subconscious level and we do them without ever thinking.

Keep a journal of what you do every week: what you eat, how you work out, what you do with your time. This way, if something is working for your weight-loss goals, you can repeat it the next week. Get the good or bad habits out of your head and down on paper so you can evaluate them. You make close to a hundred decisions a day, most of them at a subconscious level. So monitor your good and bad habits, make adjustments and allow your habits to work in your favor. Good habits would be drinking water, getting enough sleep, and getting physically active a few times a week. Bad habits would be not eating every few hours, not sleeping, and oversnacking at night.

## SELF-SABOTAGE

Sometimes people are sabotaged in their effort to lose weight by external factors, maybe friends and family who do not make healthy choices and try to lure them to stick with old habits. But sometimes it is the dieter who is uncomfortable with the changes. When you literally have to fight yourself day in and day out, it can be a tough fight; the fight of your life. I often hear people in our VIP Group say they have lost a whole lot of pounds in a couple of months but cannot see any changes in their appearance. This sense of not seeing a difference can cause you to sabotage your efforts after you have made great progress because you are not comfortable with change.

Sometimes self-sabotage is caused by issues that are more complicated than weight, such as rape, death, assault, sexual violence or abuse, abandonment. If you have deeper issues that are causing you to sabotage your success, you may want to see a therapist to gain some coping skills. All these years you could be thinking you have a problem with your weight, but the real problem is a deeper hurt or pain that you are not processing. Some of us have been using food as a coping skill for so long, we do not even realize what we are doing yet or how our habits are becoming addictive.

Dana realized through therapy that she had been so hurt in her first marriage that she felt safer being big. It was a way to push people away, especially the opposite sex. Food was attached to coping with hurt and pain, and it was a real struggle for her to give it up. She did not know how she would cope without food. If you are the kind of dieter who starts strong and then sabotages your own success, then you may need a therapist to address deeper issues and fears. Dana found her sessions to be not only helpful but an essential part of her weight-loss plan. Just as she planned her meals and physical activity, she planned her sessions with her therapist. Dana lost 115 pounds and has now maintained that weight loss for two years. She even has a new beau, who makes her laugh and smile.

Losing weight is a process that involves more than focusing on what to eat or what workouts to do. It involves dealing with inner struggles and personal issues. So many people have been trying to lose weight by following a diet or food regimen, when more than half of their challenges were internal (mental) and not physical.

# 3

---

# Stage Three—The Stall
# (The Weight-Loss Plateau)

---

E VEN WHEN YOU are on track and the pounds are melting
off, there will be a point at which your weight loss slows or
stalls. This is perfectly normal; it happens to everyone seeking
to lose weight.

I generally do not recommend tracking calories for weight
loss, but understanding how your body burns calories will help you
understand why your weight loss slows. For example, if you weigh
200 pounds, it takes 2,000 calories per day to maintain that weight.
When you drop to 180 pounds, then it will take only 1,800 calories
per day to maintain your weight. The less you weigh, the fewer
calories you need to burn to maintain your body's weight.

Therefore, when you decide to lose more and more weight,
you need to take in fewer and fewer calories. Here is what hap-

pens: At 200 pounds, you decide to take in 1,500, instead of 2,000, calories a day—a reduction of 500 calories—which will produce a weight loss of 1 pound per week. When your weight drops to 180 pounds, and you consume the same number of calories, 1,500, you are now reducing your intake by only 300 calories a day. Since you must deficit 3,500 calories to lose a pound of fat, you can see how it will take longer to lose a pound than when you weighed more. At 200 pounds, you could lose 1 pound in a week, but at 180 pounds, it will take you about twelve days to lose a pound if you continue to take in the same 1,500 calories per day.

However, do not think you can starve yourself and lose more weight. Weight loss can also slow down if you drop your calories too much, because the body thinks that it is starving. The body has a mechanism to preserve itself in case of starvation: metabolism will slow down significantly when the body senses it is getting too little food. So, ironically, at a certain point in your weight-loss journey, you do best to eat in order to lose weight.

Keep in mind that it is normal for weight loss to slow for various reasons. This can be one of the most frustrating aspects of losing weight. You put in the effort yet you do not get consistent results.

Marcy was following all the right guidance, keeping a food diary, and losing about a pound a week. She was really feeling on top of the world, as if she had found the solution to her problem. Then, after three months, she stopped losing weight for no apparent reason. Nothing had changed in her eating habits or workout routine, but her weight stayed the same for weeks. The first week, she just kept pressing; but by the second week, she felt like giving up. She said, "This always happens to me. Maybe I am not destined to be slim. I can't work this hard and not see results!"

I explained to her that losing weight was a process and that weight loss will fluctuate week to week, and sometimes the number on the scale can go up even if you have not changed your eating habits. The body is complex and will not always do what we want it to do. I went on to explain why weight loss can fluctuate throughout the week. She decided to keep pressing forward. She later lost 2 pounds in one week, after not losing any weight for an entire month. She continued losing after that. She became more patient through the process and did not quit. Just by changing her calorie intake every few days, she was able to trick her metabolism and begin losing again.

Throughout your weight-loss journey, you may actually see the number on the scale go up on some days. This is perfectly normal. Weight fluctuates due to three things in the body: water, fat, and muscle.

For many women, water is the biggest culprit, due to our hormones. Many of us gain 5 to 10 pounds of water weight during our menstrual cycle. For some, excess salt/sodium causes water to be trapped in the body tissues, making us weigh more and look bloated and puffy! So do not sweat it if your weight is a little up and down. You typically only have a problem when it is up every week, week after week!

Look into getting a Tanita scale; it will tell you your weight and the percentage of muscle, fat, and water in the body. This is helpful for people who work out!

Muscle weighs the most, more than fat, which means you can work out and build muscle and actually gain weight. But you are actually making progress by building muscle because it will help you burn fat all day long. If you are working out more than you used to and gaining muscle mass, the number on the scale might not move as much due to your gaining extra muscle. The more muscle you have, the more you will weigh, although you may be getting smaller because you have less body fat. Muscle tissue is also denser than fat tissue so although the scale may be moving slowly, rest assured that you are losing inches. You will also feel more toned, strong, and fit. If you lose muscle mass, your metabolic rate will begin to slow and you will burn fewer calories. In fact, 1 pound of fat burns about 2 calories a day to maintain itself, whereas 1 pound of lean muscle mass burns 30 to 50 calories a day to maintain itself. So just by maintaining more muscle mass, you will burn more calories throughout the day and keep your metabolism revved up. Putting on just 5 to 10 pounds of lean muscle mass will speed up your resting metabolism so you will burn more calories even when resting. So do not be afraid to work out and add more muscle as it will work to your benefit.

## 5 WAYS TO BREAK THROUGH A WEIGHT-LOSS PLATEAU

The process of breaking through a weight-loss plateau, the point at which your weight loss stalls, is mostly mental. Below I give you the five things you will need to do it.

The process of losing weight is about change, right? You are trying to do some things differently. You are trying out a new lifestyle and new eating habits. It is a process that you are trying to master. It is not, "Should I eat this or should I eat that?" It is about making the right decisions day in and day out that work in your favor. You are going to have to think about how you think about yourself, how you act, and what circumstances cause you to get off track. It takes extreme mindfulness.

### Number 1: Trick Your Metabolism by Alternating Food Intake

To prevent your body from adapting to a certain number of calories or a certain amount of food it expects to receive, it is a good idea to alternate how much food you eat each day during the week. This way you keep your metabolism constantly guessing. This means eating more food or a heavier meal a few times a week. Doing this will make your metabolism more efficient. It stays revved up in fat-burning mode. If you begin a habit of having green smoothies for breakfast and lunch and just a salad for dinner every day, that might seem like a great routine for losing weight. However, what will happen is that your body will adjust to the lower number of calories, and your metabolism will slow down in response. So, you have to mix it up and every few days, eat more than your normal meals to keep your metabolism revved up.

Everyone should have a basic understanding of how the body works with the foods we consume. You need to be aware that eating a heavier meal will probably provide you with more calories than eating a light meal. But knowing the exact calorie count is not critical to weight-loss success. Once you become aware of this, you can start listening to your body and adapting what you eat from week to week.

### Number 2: Change Up Your Workout Routine

When we move differently, the body uses different muscles, which helps to accelerate the body's natural fat-burning capabilities. Try new movement patterns or workout routines to make your workout more challenging and interesting, even if it is for less time. When we change our routines, we end up burning more calories that last well beyond the time we spend working out.

There are all kinds of fitness routines to try. Just switch them up. You can try Zumba, line-dancing, spinning, cycling, swimming, or the elliptical trainer. Try a high-intensity interval training routine, like Tabata (which takes only four minutes). There are so many ways to keep it interesting and engage new muscles that will increase your body's ability to burn fat.

### Number 3: Don't Be Impatient

It is a losing mentality to haul around 50 pounds of excess weight for ten or twenty years and then all of a sudden get mad because you have not lost 10 pounds in a month. Some of you have gotten spoiled with the 10-Day Green Smoothie Cleanse; I developed a detox program that provided fast, healthy results as detailed in my bestselling *10-Day Green Smoothie Cleanse* book. You may have lost 10 to 15 pounds in ten days and want to continue losing a pound a day. People start saying, "Oh, my, the scale is up 2 pounds. What am I going to do?"

You must press forward. You have to stay in it to win it. You are in it for the long haul.

People today have no patience; they want immediate results. With the advent of cell phones, we all essentially have a computer at our fingertips. Everything is about instant gratification. However, the reality is, when it comes to weight loss, it is a journey, a process. It probably took you years to gain weight. Do not expect to lose it all in one month.

That is too quick. It is important to understand that losing weight takes time.

If you know you are a naturally impatient person about everything, then accept that you are going to have to work very hard to be patient through this process. Normal weight loss is 1 to 2 pounds per week. That means by the end of the year—if you do not give up—you could lose anywhere from 50 to 100 pounds. Well, just think what 100 pounds looks like a year from now. Would that put you at your goal weight? Would you be in your favorite clothes again? Would you feel confident and have your sexy back? You have to keep that picture in mind, because you cannot overreact over 2 or 3 pounds when you are trying to lose 50. It requires patience.

Every time you stall, you have to mix things up. You have to do things differently to get the scale to move again. Do not be desperate for immediate results and then quit on yourself because you cannot lose 10 pounds in ten days. That is not realistic, and you need to have realistic expectations. Think about where you will be a year from now if you just stay the course.

### Number 4: Celebrate the Small Goals

I hear so many people say, "I need to lose 50 pounds." That is a great goal. But before you get to it, you need to lose the first 10 and then 10 more. How will you reward yourself at each milestone? Are you getting a pedicure? Are you buying a new outfit? What are you doing to celebrate 10? Losing 50 pounds might be a few months or even a year away, but losing 10 is within the near future. You can see it. You can feel it. Focus on the near-term small goals.

You can use a journal to write down and track your small goals. A small goal for some might be drinking alcohol only on the weekends as opposed to going to happy hour three or four times per week. I am not a big drinker, but to some people, that might be a great goal.

You know what a small goal is for me? If I am going to have a burger (no bun, of course, because I do not eat white bread), I get a side salad instead of french fries. I am pleased with myself when I do that, because I want those french fries badly! When I decide to do something that is healthier for me, it does not matter if anyone else gets excited. I am excited about the small goals.

If I do Tabata for four minutes, that is a big deal for me. After years without working out at all, four minutes is something about which I can get excited. I feel as proud as though I ran a marathon. My mind-set is to celebrate every small goal.

Do not wait to celebrate when you lose 50 pounds, celebrate when you lose 10 or 20 pounds. Maybe buy a new outfit when you hit a weight-loss milestone. Stay small in your goals. Achieve them, and then celebrate your butt off.

### Number 5: A Weight-Loss Plateau Does Not Mean You Failed

You are going to have temporary setbacks on this journey. Do not take them as a sign of a character flaw or weakness. They just mean you are human and you are just like the rest of us. So many people think, when they fall off track, even if it is for a few days, that they are just weak. Actually, they are normal because most people fall off for short periods of time. You are not weak. You are human, and all of us on this journey are having our days and weeks in which we're just messing up.

If you eat a piece of cake and feel like, "Oh, I shouldn't have had a piece of cake," do not lose focus, throw up your hands, and devour the whole cake. A piece of cake is fine. Enjoy it. Do not say, "I am so weak." You are not weak. You are just like the rest of us, and we are all going through the same thing. We are all having the same struggle. The people who win are the ones who pick up the next day, press forward, and try their best to do better than they did the day before. And even if they do not, they try again. You only lose when you give up!

Next time you are tempted to quit and try a fad diet or magic weight-loss pill, remember why you started and keep going. Celebrate the journey. The journey to permanent weight loss is filled with both joy and frustration. Yes, we can all agree that it is frustrating to put in the effort and not see results. However, your ability to press forward and continue will ultimately determine if you will be a successful "loser" (really a winner) in the end. If you can learn to appreciate the process along the way, your journey will be that much more doable and rewarding. Weight loss takes time, energy, and focus.

# 4

---

# Stage Four—Reaching Your
# Ideal Weight

---

CAN RECALL TWO times in my life, in my twenties and again in my thirties, where I gained 38 and 40 pounds respectively and I tried several diets and was very committed to losing weight. I followed all the typical advice to "eat less and exercise more" but it just didn't work for me. So, being a nutritionist, I designed a weight-loss system that has helped me and my clients shed pounds fast. I was able to go from a size 16 to a size 6. The day I got back into my skinny jeans, I jumped for joy as if I had won the lottery. Getting back down to the size I was in my early twenties felt amazing. It was such an important goal for me. I had worked so hard to learn what was causing my stubborn body fat, and my efforts paid off. I had a feeling of accomplishment, joy, and pride. I could not wait to celebrate with my family and friends who had supported me along the way.

I have personally watched hundreds of individuals not just lose weight but also get to their ideal weight. Kiana decided to lose 50 pounds before her fortieth birthday. She remained steadfast and was very successful. She hit her goal weight of 140 pounds and looked and felt great. She received much attention, praise, and support, for those who knew her well knew how much of a struggle it had been for her. Kiana described the feeling of getting to her goal weight as one of exhilaration and exuberance. She marveled at her new dress size, her figure from the side, and how people treated her once she was at her goal weight.

She savored all the benefits of her new size, like being able to cross her legs and not having to hide her belly when she sat down. This feeling of accomplishment motivated her to maintain her goal weight. She would run into people who were totally shocked by her transformation, and that kept her going as well. Her favorite compliment was "Girl, you look fabulous! You have lost a lot of weight!" This feedback was so motivating that each day she woke up and remained mindful of what she ate and how often she worked out. Kiana said she stayed on this high for three or four months after she reached her goal weight. She knew to keep up with the regimen that got her there and monitor her activities every day. After all, she did not want to let down so many people that she had inspired.

## TIME TO ENJOY THE NEW YOU

Believe it or not, many people have a hard time adjusting to being thin. Just as we did not accept it when we were overweight, we may also struggle to accept that we are now slim. Our self-image does not always change just because we lose weight. I have lost four dress sizes over the past decade and yet I still see fat on my hips, thighs, and butt. If you called yourself fat, fluffy, or chubby, you will likely continue to see yourself that way for some time. Even though you know you are no longer overweight, in your head you are still the fat girl or chubby friend.

When you become aware of this feeling of thinking of yourself as chubby even though you are not, this is a good time to take "after" photos so you can see your success. When you see yourself in a photo, there is a no way to deny what you look like.

Shopping for clothes and buying smaller sizes is another way to help you see your success. If you buy a size 6 or 8, you know for certain that you are far from overweight. That is confirmation that you have achieved weight-loss success.

## WHEN THE HONEYMOON FADES

I personally have never met anyone who stayed the exact same size every day for a lifetime. Once you have maintained your weight loss for several months, the high will start to wear off. You might even gain a few (5 to 10) pounds back. Friends and family are used to your new size, so the compliments become less frequent. You begin getting weary of maintaining your weight and all that that entails: eating right, working out, and just being aware of what you put into your body.

After six months, Kiana began to gain some of her weight, about 15 pounds, back. Now she was no longer receiving so many compliments. She could no longer wear her new smaller sizes and was starting to feel defeated.

This is a very tricky stage in the weight-loss journey. Slight weight regain, if not managed properly, can send people on a downward spiral that leads them back to their heaviest weight. The reality is that you can expect some weight gain, but the trick is to be able to lose that weight before it spirals out of control. To do that, you have to deal with the emotions that come along with weight regain.

When you start to gain the weight back, you may feel sad, shameful, and dejected. If you expect this to happen, you stand a much better chance of not spiraling out of control. You become aware that this is the process, this is a typical experience, and you are just like other successful folks who have lost weight. Learning to work your weight back down after gaining a few pounds back is a critical part of learning how to keep your weight off permanently.

Kiana's mind started to play tricks on her. She started thinking, "I don't want to have to work this hard to maintain my weight. I still look good because I'm still not as overweight as I was." Kiana began to forget how unhappy she had been at her highest weight.

It is important to appreciate your new body every day. You have to remind yourself how great you felt and looked at your goal weight. You have to remember how much energy you had, how good your sleep was, and how you have fewer aches and pains. You have to remind yourself that you deserve to be healthy, happy, and fit. You have to remind yourself that it is worth it.

## WHAT TO EXPECT DURING THIS STAGE

The timing of this stage is usually somewhere between six months to a year into maintaining your weight. This is the point where the high is gone and the compliments have stopped coming. The work of being mindful of what you eat, working out, keeping a food diary also seems tedious and boring, like a chore. This is the time to acknowledge these feelings for what they are, which is very normal.

Kiana had stopped making her green smoothies, (She had been following the Green Smoothie Cleanse which yields fast, healthy weight loss using green smoothies as a primary meal every day). She stopped taking her lunch to work, and was easily stressed. She even started buying unhealthy snacks from the grocery store, telling herself she would snack in moderation. But her snacking got out of control again. She regained 30 of the 50 pounds she had lost. Nevertheless, after dealing with the initial disappointment and shame, she dusted herself off and got back on track.

Every day, you face a slippery slope that will determine your ultimate success or failure. You will want to eat a "cheat meal" more often and will tell yourself that you deserve an ice cream sundae. It is not that you cannot have one from time to time, but this is not the time to indulge in an ice cream sundae every day. The old behavior of using food to deal with feelings of sadness has to remain in the past.

If you used food to cope with loneliness, sadness, fear, anger, or boredom, remember that this book will teach you coping skills to address these feelings in the future. You must remember the new and better ways of dealing with the issues that come up in your life. It is your job to come up with new solutions to deal with life situations. For example, if you eat out of boredom and loneliness at night, get out of the house and go have some fun. Go to a Zumba class or take a salsa dance class. Come up with a list of things to do, either in or out of the house, that will keep you busy and having fun. Always remind yourself of how far you have come, and although you have had a small setback, you can still press forward and win this weight-loss battle once and for all.

Kiana is still in the game and weighing herself every day. She lost control of her eating for a few months but got back on track by getting physically active, increasing her detox methods each week, drinking water consistently, and adjusting her calorie intake every few days. She was able to turn things around because she knew her setback was temporary. As hard as it was for her to deal with weight regain, she began to realize that this was a lifelong journey and that she had better tools in her tool kit.

# 5

## Stage Five—Maintaining (Keeping the Weight Off)

I N THIS FINAL stage of the five stages of weight loss, you successfully changed the majority of your bad habits and have lived a healthy lifestyle for a year or more. In this stage, you begin to acknowledge that you truly do live life differently. You realize that foods have no power over you and you do not even desire or crave them regularly. You know how harmful bad eating was to your health and weight and you do not need the temporary fulfillment that emotional eating provided you.

You walk around with a new confidence because your body has undergone a complete transformation. People often ask you how you did it; you are a walking inspiration and receive compliments on a regular basis. Let me also say "Congratulations!" for making the lifestyle change for good. You now know this new healthy lifestyle is just as easy to live as the unhealthy life you lived in the past.

To ensure that you understand what I mean by "lifestyle change," I want to take a moment to explain this further. First, you really have to forget about dieting! Typically, you "go on" a diet, which implies that at some point you "go off" the diet. A typical diet is something you do for a specified period of time. However, what typically happens when you "go off" the diet? You gain all the weight back. With a lifestyle change, you are changing your eating habits and you naturally desire and crave healthier foods, so you never have to think about dieting again. In this phase, you actually forget about dieting and change the way and style in which you live.

I believe maintenance is one of the most important stages of the weight-loss journey. Learning to keep the weight off is the key to success and where the majority of people struggle. In fact, about 90 percent of people who lose weight on a diet gain the weight back in three to five years. While no one wants to lose a lot of weight, get all the compliments, and then turn around and gain it all back, it happens every day. Permanent weight loss will be determined in this phase. People are often surprised by the fact that the work does not end in this phase. They think they will reach their weight-loss goal and then be done. You need to be smarter than that. Know that to maintain the weight loss will require as much work as losing it.

## WHO IS SUCCESSFUL AT MAINTAINING WEIGHT LOSS?

So what sets apart those who are successful at losing weight and keeping it off from those who do not? The thousands of clients I have worked with have taught me a lot about what it takes to lose weight permanently. Part 2 of this book, "Seven Mental

Strategies for Weight-Loss Success," provides strategies that successful weight-losers employ to keep the weight off.

One thing these successful "losers" have in common is a recognition that they have made a lifestyle change, adopted a different mind-set. They eat a certain way each week, but they no longer "diet." They can have a cheat meal from time to time, but they get right back on track swiftly and consistently. That is what it means to make a lifestyle change. This is the new you, this is how you live.

Furthermore, they all struggled in the first two years of weight maintenance, but once they got past that, they were all successful at keeping the weight off for years and even decades. Weight regain typically happens within the first two years. This is important to understand. If you have lost and gained weight repeatedly, you should expect to struggle in the first year or two after you lose weight. Know that this is normal and get mentally prepared for the struggle. Give yourself time to adjust through this process. Over 75 percent of the successful ones say it got easier over time and the longer you keep the weight off, the less likely it is to come back.

## WEIGHT REGAIN

Be realistic in your expectations. Maintaining your weight does not mean you will stay at the exact same weight week after week, month after month. During weight maintenance, you gain and lose small amounts (5 to 10 pounds) all the time. Ideally, you must come up with a weight range in which you live comfortably. For some it is a range of 3 to 5 pounds to ensure that they do not let the weight spiral out of control.

The first two years in this weight-maintenance stage are critical in predicting long-term success. Those who go past their comfortable weight range begin to struggle to get back to their ideal weight that they had once achieved. This is why focus and work is still required in this stage.

The reason you should allow for a comfortable weight range to lose and gain weight is because weight gain can come out of nowhere. Weight regain is almost inevitable, so be prepared to deal with it. If you are thinking you will not gain any weight during this stage, it can take you mentally off track when you take on a few pounds. It is always best to be mentally prepared to fight to maintain the weight-loss success you worked so hard to achieve.

When your weight goes higher than your upper limit, you have to buckle down and get back to the habits that helped you lose weight in the first place (see more on habits in chapter 10) Were you part of a support group? Did you have coping skills to avoid emotional eating? Did you work out more regularly? Putting those behaviors and habits into practice makes it relatively easy to get back down to your ideal weight.

Monitor your weight regularly. Stay aware. Take the small weight gains within your acceptable range in stride. It is not a matter of obsessing over the scale, weighing yourself multiple times per day. The day-by-day weight fluctuations are not important in the big picture. When I hear folks complain about gaining 2 to 3 pounds, I know they are not prepared for the small weight fluctuations that will come.

If you want to weigh yourself once a day, do it first thing in the morning so that you can get a consistent read each day. Many people choose to weigh themselves weekly so they do not obsess about the numbers on a daily basis, and this is also fine.

Many folks are so discouraged by the scale that it leads them to be frustrated and then to give up. It is important that you understand what is happening on your weight-loss journey. We want our weight simply to give us a clear picture and not send us off the deep end. Keeping track will alert you to when you need to make adjustments on your journey.

Do not use unreasonable methods to lose weight or to get to an especially low weight that will be too hard to maintain. If it required unrealistic behaviors to get to that weight, then to maintain it will make your life unbearable. You want a realistic weight that you can actually maintain and still enjoy life. Many of us would love to be the weight we were in college, but to get to and maintain that weight would require an unreasonable amount of effort week to week.

Find the weight that you can accept and maintain and you will be much happier in this place. Find a comfortable weight at which you can love and accept yourself. Once you find a good maintenance weight, know that it is a lifelong journey. In addition, know that there are few things in life that can give you such a feeling of accomplishment. Own your success, give yourself credit, and enjoy your new weight.

Yes, the weight-loss phase has its own challenges, but keeping the weight off just brings new challenges. The goal of this book is to help you be fully equipped for the challenges at each stage.

## BE PREPARED FOR BOREDOM AND DISAPPOINTMENT

One of the greatest obstacles for maintaining weight loss is boredom. Compared to the thrill of losing weight and getting all the compliments, this phase can feel somewhat dull. Tammy lost over 125 pounds by eating clean, that is, eating whole, real foods, and exercising. After being consistent on her journey for so long, she became bored with her routine. However, she realized that this was a lifestyle change and this was a normal feeling. She continued to put in the work. She did not use fad diets or magic weight-loss pills. She is a changed person who simply eats well and makes physical movement a regular part of her routine. She established many new habits and behaviors. She knew these behaviors were how she lost the weight in the first place. She knows what to do to stay there. When you create new behaviors and habits, you have the foundation you need to ease into maintenance.

The tedious nature of maintaining weight loss can get dull and boring, so this is the time to remain as vigilant and focused as ever.

Many times when people lose weight, they expect great things to come their way, like love. They always believed that if they just lost weight, they would find love or the spouse that had eluded them. While this may happen, sometimes it does not. Finding love is a challenge for many people, even for those who are not overweight.

Understand too that family relationships and friendships can change for the better or for the worse. When you improve your life, not everyone will be happy with you or for you. People generally do not like change and most of your friends or family may have always known you as the overweight one. They are comfortable with you playing your role. They may have a hard time adjusting to the new you. We assume that everyone will be happy about our weight loss. And some are. Some friends and family, however, may actually feel threatened by your new success, your new body, your new confidence and new attention that you are getting. Some people will be genuinely happy and some will be threatened. Know that those who really love you will adjust to the new you in time.

## BUT I'M STILL NOT SKINNY!

People who lose weight often simply cannot see it when they look in the mirror. It will be important to look at photos of yourself to help convince yourself of how great you look. It may take some time to see your weight-loss success. You may get to a point where you do not see yourself as overweight but still feel that you are just not thin enough. This is something to plan for so that you do not get disappointed when you reach your goal weight. People are constantly telling you how great you look, but you look in the mirror and see something else. This is normal, especially for those who have been overweight for many years. Our self-image is that we are overweight and it becomes difficult to change how we see ourselves. This is why it is also important to keep a list of nonscale-related benefits, such as better sleep, fewer aches and pains, lower cholesterol, increased energy, and clearer skin. Anything that helps to reinforce your feeling of success is crucial during this stage. Our self-image gets set somewhere along the way, and it is very difficult to change it.

If you have done the hard work and succeeded at losing weight, celebrate your success. Congratulate yourself. Take all the credit for it because it is hard work and your body has rewarded you for your efforts. Weight loss was not given to you, it was earned by you. It took a lot of focus and determination.

## DON'T TAKE A VACATION FROM HEALTHY LIVING

Linda lost 65 pounds and maintained it for over a year. Then her family decided to take a vacation in the mountains for an entire month. Unfortunately, she did not just take a vacation from work but also from all the habits and behaviors that had helped her maintain a healthy lifestyle. She failed to make sound eating decisions and indulged in desserts every night. Linda enjoyed a break from real life and everything that came along with her life. It was as though she went on a binge, eating anything and everything.

At the end of the vacation, she came back 10 pounds heavier. Then she had to work like crazy just to reestablish her good eating habits and behaviors. It took her about three to four months to work her way down to her comfortable maintenance weight. She found it incredibly time-consuming and difficult to lose those 10 pounds and felt like she had set herself back too far. So she decided she would never again take a vacation from healthy eating just because she was on vacation.

Enjoying a few cheat meals on a vacation is fine, but reverting to the entire old lifestyle is a very self-defeating choice. You can enjoy vacations and holidays without overeating and indulging and still feel good when you return and just continue on your lifestyle of maintaining your weight.

Forget about your old habits, as they will always lead you back to your unhealthy weight. The more people understand this, the more they will stop losing and gaining over and over again. Once you learn how to lose weight, you can maintain and enjoy your healthy, slim body. You may miss some of your old comfort foods, but they are still there to enjoy from time to time—just do not let them become a habit. Stay the course. It is so worth it!

# Part Two

---

# THE SOLUTIONS: SEVEN MENTAL STRATEGIES FOR WEIGHT-LOSS SUCCESS

"The Solutions: Seven Mental Strategies for Weight-Loss Success," introduces the SUCCESS System, which teaches you seven new mental strategies, habits, and approaches to permanent weight loss. Some of the seven strategies will be more applicable to you and your current journey than others, but the more you apply, the better your results will be.

1. *SLAY Resistance: Stop Procrastination Once and For All.* Learn how to slay resistance, the most toxic force in the world. Resistance is that lethargic or apathetic feeling of not wanting to do something you know is good for you. Resistance causes us to procrastinate or delay starting something that is good for us. You must slay resistance in order to achieve the success you desire.

2. *USE VISUALIZATION: Use Visualization Techniques for Weight Loss.* An effective approach to losing weight permanently is to use visualization to get your mind and body to work together to get slim. Folks have had amazing results with visualization techniques without having to starve themselves or deprive the body in any way. Visualization is a mind-body approach that makes permanent weight loss easy and sustainable. I will teach you how to allow your mind to work with your body to transform yourself from the inside out.

3. *COMMIT: Learn How to Commit to Losing Weight.* Are you merely interested in losing weight or are you committed to losing weight? If you are truly committed, you will do what it takes and make the necessary sacrifices to lose weight. People fail not because of lack

of interest or desire but because of lack of commitment. Learn the different types of motivation and how to apply them to your journey.

4. *CONTROL EMOTIONS: Don't Eat Your Heart Out.* Learn the signals (such as boredom, depression, loneliness, frustration, anger) that trigger emotional eating. These are the wake-up calls that let us know we are dealing with toxic emotions that need to be processed and managed.

5. *ESTABLISH SUCCESS HABITS: Design Your Life for Weight-Loss Success.* You cannot rely on willpower and self-control to lose weight—you have to control your environment and circumstances. Your ability to maintain self-control will depend on your environment. If your house is hectic and chaotic, or if you are stressed or in a bad mood or easily distracted, you will struggle to maintain self-control. All of these circumstances can happen each and every day, so in order to have more self-control, you will have to change your environment by establishing success habits.

6. *SUPPORT FROM OTHERS: Have a Support System in Place.* Studies show that those who have a support community have more long-term success with weight loss. Learn how to create support systems and accountability partners.

7. *SUPERCHARGE YOUR SPIRITUAL LIFE: Tap into Your Spiritual Power to Achieve Weight-Loss Success.* Until your mind and spirit are engaged in your weight-loss efforts, excess weight will continue to be a problem for you. The ultimate problem is not your physical weight but what is happening in your mind and spirit causing you to gain weight.

# 6

## SLAY Resistance

Tomorrow is the day you have decided that you are going to wake up early and begin to exercise regularly. You set your alarm for 5:00 a.m. so you can go to the gym before work. You fall asleep. The alarm clock loudly goes off letting you know it is time to get out of bed. You are now confronted with your first decision of the day. Will you get up or will you hit the snooze button? You decide to press the snooze button and go back to sleep. Is this a big deal? You best believe it is. You just lost the first battle of the day. You had decided to set the alarm early so you could get up and work out, but instead you hit the snooze and went back to sleep. What just happened? Resistance just won. Resistance has beaten you before you even got out of bed. You now have an uphill battle for the rest of the day.

Most of us have two lives, the unlived life and the actual one we live day to day. Between the two lives stands resistance. The unlived life is where all of our hopes, dreams, goals, and heart's desires are, which is often different from the life, career, and home where we actually live day to day. I have been battling resistance my whole life and I imagine you have too. What is resistance? In my opinion, resistance is one of the most toxic forces in the world. Resistance is that lethargic or apathetic feeling of not wanting to do something you know is good for you. Resistance causes us to procrastinate, or delay starting something that is good for us. Do you constantly set goals and not accomplish them? Well, resistance is the reason you have not achieved the success you desired.

To give in to resistance weakens the spirit and stunts our growth and makes us not be who we were born to be. You may not have taken the time to name this lethargic, apathetic feeling, but chances are you have come face to face with resistance every day. Resistance is there, preventing you from living your best life.

Resistance cannot be seen, heard, or touched, but it can most definitely be felt. Resistance is the enemy within. Resistance has many masks: fear, procrastination, fatigue, doubt, indecision, laziness, self-sabotage, and pride. As a general rule of thumb, the greater the calling on your life, the stronger the resistance. Our genius, our gifts, our talents, and our purpose for being on this earth are on the other side of resistance. You have to fight through resistance in the smallest tasks of the day to fulfill your life's goals.

I struggle with resistance every day. When I sit down to write, I immediately procrastinate by picking up my phone to see what is going on on Facebook or to check email. This is what resistance looks like for me. I have written several *New*

*York Times* bestselling books, but every time I sit down to write, I will have to slay resistance just to get started. Resistance is subtle yet so powerful. It will stop you in your tracks if you do not recognize it and defeat it each time. How many people have tried to write a book but never finished it? How many people have tried to lose weight but never achieved their weight-loss goal? Why? Resistance has defeated them and most of the time they didn't even realize it. Do you not believe me? I want you to stop and think about it right now. How many times did you say you were going to workout or start a new diet, and you simply did not do it, day after day, week after week? Resistance is real. Resistance is burying you and your dreams each and every day.

## TAKE ACTION

Resistance will make you feel discouraged and want to quit. Resistance will make you feel hopeless about changing things in your life. Do not give in to discouragement. Do not let fear paralyze you. Resistance can start out as unhappiness but quickly turn to self-hate or even worse, depression or dysfunctional behavior. You have to focus on things that give you the spiritual fortitude to fight through and continue pursuing your best life. For me, I turn to God in prayer and simply take some small action toward my goal each day to slay resistance. Some days it's drinking more water, sometimes it's doing a hundred squats or simply walking to clear my mind and plan for the next day.

Think of resistance as a wall that you have to break down in order to start something new.

Taking action helps. Think of one thing, one positive action you can take this week to slay resistance. Maybe it begins with telling someone, "I am unhappy. I feel discouraged." Just by acknowledging it, you begin to cast out fear and hopelessness. Decide today that you will take one action, no matter how small, that will help break through resistance. I do not mean start pretending to be happy or being dishonest with yourself. I mean acknowledge your unhappiness, as that dissatisfaction that is leading you to something different, brand new, or greater. It is your wake-up call to listen to what your Spirit is trying to say.

Pay more attention to the quiet discontent in your life. Do not try to cover it up with money, sex, people, drugs, or alcohol. Those things are distractions that will just keep you too busy to achieve the one thing you desire in your life.

## CREATE NEW HABITS

Our habits, the things we do day in and day out, have a major impact on our lives. They shape our entire future and destiny. Resistance thrives when you have bad habits. What bad habits have you picked up to avoid doing the hard work of your life?

Let us think about some of your habits and daily routines. Do you spend time in prayer or self-reflection in the morning? Do you walk the dog? Do you eat the same thing for breakfast? Do you read a book before bed? These daily habits and routines create the rhythms of your life. Yet when was the last time you deliberately established a routine to create a life-altering habit. We will have to change our habits and routine or else we are going to fight resistance over fifty times a day. If every time you get frustrated, mad, lonely, bored, or tired and do not have a habit or routine to sustain you, you will just give in to resistance.

Most highly successful people have better habits than most of us do. Their habits consistently make it easier to defeat resistance. Good habits will help us defeat resistance in our lives as well.

## CLEAN UP THE MESSES IN YOUR LIFE

Resistance thrives in messiness. We all have messes in our lives. Home mess. Relationship mess. Work mess. Kid mess. Some messes are small, some are life-altering. Sickness and death, disease and heartbreak, fear and pain, abuse and addiction, disappointment and failure, injustice and shattered dreams—all of these things make life very messy. Doctors estimate that 70 percent to 80 percent of their business is nonhealth-related. People are not actually sick; they are just living a messy life.

When I was younger, in my twenties, I had no idea that life was so messy. This probably worked in my favor because if I had known as a young person how challenging, heartbreaking, and messy life could be, I might have thrown in the towel.

Even though life is messy, it does not mean we just live a life of messiness. We do not have to let the mess define us. We are equipped and capable of doing something about it. We have to confront our own mess, and how we have contributed to it, as well as take responsibility for the mess we have caused in other people's lives. We are here to put in the work of eliminating messiness, fighting the good fight, and living our very best life.

Everyone is fighting the good fight against some type of internal struggle. What battle are you struggling with right now? What battle is your spouse or loved one struggling with? When you acknowledge that others are also fighting a hard battle, you can rise to the occasion to help them through it. If someone is nasty, rude, or mean to you, just know he or she may be going through something difficult. Do not treat them the way they are treating you, because criticism and cruelty harms others. Rise to the occasion and allow the greatest part of your being to show them compassion and love. When we all do this, collectively we all win against a messy life.

Show compassion and love to everyone by simply greeting someone with a smile, praying for them, and showing them more love than they deserve.

## ENHANCE YOUR SPIRITUAL LIFE

So many of us focus on getting physically healthy. But what about spiritual health?

When was the last time you paused to think deeply about your life and your happiness? The quality of the life you are living? Most people do not think about their lives this way because they are simply trying to muster up enough energy to get through their busy, hectic day. They are struggling through each week, trying to make it to the weekend when they can just chill or do something fun. They simply have become indifferent and have lost hope for getting to the next level in life. When was the last time you purposefully thought about the life you are living? Are you spiritually healthy? Are you walking in purpose and winning day-to-day battles? Are you slaying resistance and staying focused and motivated? Are you living your best life—physically, emotionally, and spiritually?

Answer this question: How is your prayer life? Just as your blood pressure is a great indicator of your physical health, your prayer life is a great barometer of your spiritual health. Taking stock of your prayer life will allow you to get more in sync with your spiritual needs. It will help you get to the root of your cravings—not just your physical cravings, but your soul cravings.

Place the Word of God or inspirational books where they are visible to you every day and spend more time reading and strengthening your spiritual life.

## FIVE MINUTES A DAY TO SLAY RESISTANCE

There is a phrase that church folks say: Prayer changes everything. It is the truth. In fact, nothing ever really changes until we give daily prayer a place in our lives. Take five minutes each day to pray with God. If you do not believe in praying to God, then still take five minutes a day to reflect on your current struggles and challenges and think about the best direction for your current situation. I am asking you to take five minutes out of your day to make prayer or self-reflection a daily habit. Put Post-it notes throughout your home or car until you remember this daily habit. By doing this, you are slaying resistance each day.

Resistance will try to keep you from this quiet time every day. Resistance will encourage you to do it later. But you can seize control by taking time each morning to begin your day in prayer or self-reflection.

The five-minute daily habit of prayer or self-reflection leads to spiritual health. The more we do this, the clearer our direction becomes in our life. Five minutes a day is a simple and achievable task. Try it daily and watch your life change for the better.

## CONCLUSION

We all have a bit of spiritual laziness that causes us to have a weak mind that cannot defeat resistance. It is important to have a strong mind and spirit that thrives and shines bright in a world full of hopelessness. I am confident that five minutes a day of prayer or self-reflection will help you create some powerful spiritual experiences that yield amazing results in your life.

As you continue on your spiritual journey, be watchful for the resistance that has defeated you in the past. Be observant. Guard against cynics and critics. Resistance will use them to discourage you or distract you from living your best life. Stay focused on your life's calling and purpose. Resistance is the only thing standing between you and the happiness you desire. Watch for the resistance, recognize it, and fight against it, and it will lose its power over you with time. Each time you break through resistance, you are moving toward the life you imagined for yourself since you were born.

# 7

## Use Visualization Techniques for Weight Loss

YOU ARE READING this because you probably have tried to lose weight in the past and it did not work. You may think you failed at dieting or wasted time with gym memberships. You may be feeling disappointed in yourself.

Before we go any further, let us be sure you understand something: You did not fail on those diets, those diets failed you. Dieting does not work because it does not address the underlying reasons we gain weight in the first place. Sure, you can force yourself to lose weight temporarily by eating less or avoiding unhealthy foods, but like so many other dieters, you will always gain the weight back. You generally can keep up with healthy eating and exercising for a while, but eventually you veer off track and give in to the foods you crave. You have to get to the root of the problem that causes the cravings for unhealthy foods. Rather than continuing this losing battle with dieting, it is time to focus on changing the way you think to solve your weight problems once and for all.

An effective approach to losing weight permanently is to use visualization to get your mind and body to work together. Folks have had amazing results with visualization without having to starve themselves or deprive their body in any way. Visualization is a mind-body approach that makes permanent weight loss easier and sustainable. I will teach you how to allow your mind to work with your body to transform yourself from the inside out.

Hundreds of thousands of people have used visualization methods to achieve dramatic weight loss. These people dieted on and off for years, but are now slimmer and healthier and no longer at war with their bodies. I am not saying they are perfect, as they do have cheat meals and sometimes lose their motivation, but they have found a way to achieve their weight goals and then maintain them.

Visualization only takes a few minutes a day, and doing it daily will yield tremendous benefits. The more you practice, the better you will get over time.

## HOW VISUALIZATION WORKS TO HELP YOU LOSE WEIGHT

Leptin is the master hormone in charge of body weight. Leptin controls how hungry you are on a daily basis. When leptin does not function properly, it creates an imbalance that results in a slow metabolism, premature aging, and disease. Many obese and overweight people have a hormonal condition called leptin resistance. This means that the brain is no longer listening to the hormone leptin, which is the same as having no leptin at all; and they just get fatter and fatter. The fat cells fail to respond to leptin's message. Leptin resistance disrupts the body's natural ability to regulate appetite and metabolism. If you become leptin-resistant, you will eat and eat as if you are starving. Some people get extremely obese because their bodies never receive the message to stop eating and start burning.

Once you understand leptin resistance, it makes sense why restrictive dieting (extreme reduction in calories) does not work. Restrictive dieting mimics a famine. As you starve yourself and fight your cravings, your body thinks you are in an actual famine; your survival mechanisms kick in and you become leptin-resistant. This causes you to be hungry and tired all the time.

When you practice visualizations, you can rewire your brain and reduce the inflammatory hormones that cause leptin resistance. You will stop craving unhealthy junk foods and desire real foods. You will have a balanced body chemistry that will cause you to desire nutrient-rich foods that fuel the body for healthy weight loss.

Visualization is like having a conversation with your brain, sending signals to your body that you are not in a famine state and that you've got plenty to eat and don't need the extra weight on your body. This allows your body to release the weight naturally. When you unlock the secrets of communicating with your brain, the health and fitness possibilities are endless.

There are five steps to mastering visualization to help accelerate weight loss. Let us examine them.

## FIVE STEPS TO USING VISUALIZATION
## FOR WEIGHT LOSS

### Step 1: Prep the Mind

Proper posture is critical for visualization. Sit up straight in a comfortable chair and clasp your hands loosely together in your lap. Be sure to straighten your spine and keep it straight throughout your visualization.

Focus your breathing through your nose with your mouth closed.

Now you want to bring awareness into your body and be present in the moment. You can achieve this by praying, journaling, stretching, painting, taking a hot bath, doing yoga, or listening to relaxing music. Then you want to find pictures or images that immediately make you relax. Use these to help you get your mind into a relaxed state. For some, it could be an image of loved ones or family members. You might simply look at a white light. It is a good idea to try a few images to determine which ones relax you as soon as you see them.

### Step 2: Create Positive Affirmations

Now that you are present in the moment, it is time to start communicating to your mind. You can use positive affirmations to create the change you desire in your life, such as losing weight or quitting smoking. Now be aware of every cell in your body and imagine every cell glowing with white light.

Since we are focusing on weight loss, here are some positive affirmations that focus on the change you want to create in your life. You should repeat these affirmations for two minutes daily so that every cell in your body can imagine them.

1. *I love myself.* I am not ashamed of my body, for it is just the house for my spiritual and mental self; it does not define my true self.
2. *I have a loving relationship with food.* I know that food is a gift from God that I am grateful for because it nourishes my body.
3. *I am thankful for my body* and look forward to a slimmer, healthier body as I become more enlightened about healthy eating.
4. *I am not afraid to get on the scale* because the number that I weigh is not as important as the overall healthiness of my body. A healthy body is a beautiful body.
5. *I forgive myself and other people.* No more arguing and fighting, only letting go of stresses, failures, and disappointments.

### Step 3: Release the Weight

Now it is time to envision the weight melting off your body. Visualize the fat being released from your body and imagine your body getting slimmer and slimmer. Think of the excess fat being sucked away from your body. If you think of the fat as energy, imagine the fat releasing into a whirlpool until it disappears. Imagine the excess fat on your stomach, legs, hips, arms, chest, neck, and face all getting sucked into a whirlpool until it disappears. Visualize yourself sitting still with no excess fat on your body.

### Step 4: Picture Your Ideal Body

Now that the fat has melted away, create a picture of your ideal body. Think of your desired shape—your waistline, breasts, arms, and legs. Think about how you would feel sitting in this body shape. Are your muscles tight, is your stomach flat, is your booty toned? Truly imagine what it feels like to have this ideal body shape.

Now picture going to work with this ideal body and what your friends and coworkers would say to you. Imagine how your spouse/partner would look at you with this ideal shape. Can you see yourself on the beach or on a date with this ideal body? As you go through all these scenarios, be as specific as possible. Imagine the conversation with your friends and family when they see your ideal body. What exact words would each of them say? If you were on the beach in a bikini, can you feel the wind blowing through your hair and the sand on your feet?

Create these visuals of your ideal body shape and feel what your life would be like, both personally and professionally.

### Step 5: Envision Your Future

Visualize what you want your life to look like in the future. See yourself becoming slimmer, fitter, and healthier day by day, month by month. Envision getting promoted and finding more career opportunities down the road. See yourself marrying the love of your life or finding your ideal mate. Envision all the chronic health issues disappearing—no more high blood pressure, inflammation, or high cholesterol. See your health and weight issues receding into the past.

See your ideal body shape pulling you toward more love, better health, greater career opportunities, and total success in life. Imagine achieving all your life goals effortlessly. You make the right food choices, the right decisions at work, and the best decisions in your love life. Let your thoughts pull you like a magnet to your perfect, healthy, and successful life. Whether it is success in weight loss, career, relationships, or whatever you have ever dreamed for your life, allow the picture of your beautiful future to fill your mind, body, and soul. Then, before you open your eyes, with the power of your mind, say, "I have created my ideal body and my successful life."

If you feel like it, you can stay still for a few more minutes focusing on your breathing or you can open your eyes and end the visualization. This five-step visualization should take five to seven minutes each day, from beginning to end.

## VISUALIZATION EXERCISES FOR SPECIFIC GOALS (OPTIONAL EXERCISES)

The visualization exercises below will help you target specific situations or addictions that you want to address in your life. It does not matter which you choose or what order you do them in, as they can be customized based upon your specific needs. However, repetition is key. *If you identify a few visualization exercises you want to do, be sure to do them daily for at least a week to implant the actions in your mind and body.* As long as you stay consistent, visualizing your perfect life and body, you will move toward achieving those things. Read them aloud and feel and embrace the following visualization exercises.

## #1 Love Your Body

Imagine every cell of your body being draped with love. From head to toe, feel your body being charged with a beautiful ray of light that flows through every cell. You can feel negativity, darkness, and fear all get replaced with love. Imagine your heart filling with a loving energy flowing through your blood to every cell and tissue in your body. Say aloud, "I am love. I love myself. I am loved. I feel love. I am grateful for the love in my life. I am thankful for those who love me. Every part of my body is being healed with love." Know that the power of love is perfect, healthy, all-knowing, self-healing, and abundant.

Imagine the white light getting brighter and brighter as you embrace more love within your body. You feel tremendous love from God throughout your body. You feel tremendous love and support from family and friends. Everywhere you look, you see and feel love. Everywhere you turn, you feel loved, protected, and appreciated from everyone you know. You send a signal to everyone who knows you that you are to be recognized, celebrated, appreciated, and loved. You see yourself talking to people and radiating love to the point that they want to embrace you. They notice how beautiful, loving, and radiant you are. Your spouse or significant other is so loving toward you and you embrace all the love they have for you. You radiate love, you generate love, and you bask in the beautiful glow of love!

## #2 Release the Weight

Imagine all the excess weight on your body turning into liquid and evaporating from your body. Imagine excess fat being sucked into a whirlpool and completely disappearing. Imagine the excess fat on your face, arms, stomach, and legs all getting sucked into a whirlpool away from your body. You then look at your body and realize it is thin—the ideal shape you have always dreamed of. All the excess body fat is gone for good. Take a moment to feel what it is like to be at your ideal shape.

As every day passes, you get thinner, healthier, more fit and toned. You are the picture of health. You have energy, vitality, and radiant skin. You see yourself in new clothes for your ideal body. You have released the excess weight from your body and are on an incredible high of excitement and joy.

When you are ready, open your eyes, feeling confident that you have made a positive change toward becoming slimmer, fitter, and healthier. Embrace a more successful, joyful life with effortless weight loss that will last for a lifetime.

### #3 Become Vibrant and Healthy

Imagine every cell in your body saying, "I feel healthy, alive, radiant, fit, and vibrant. I am nourished. I am satisfied. I feel complete in my life right now." Imagine every cell in your body healed and healthy and all excess fat removed from your body. All the excess fat has disappeared, never to be seen again, and you feel energetic and healthy in your ideal weight. Imagine yourself walking outside with pep in your step. You feel totally nourished, and complete.

Imagine yourself eating foods that fuel and energize your body. High-nutrient foods cause your skin to glow and make you look younger than your age. Envision yourself craving whole, natural, nutrient-dense foods that make you feel nourished and satisfied. With every bite of food, your body gets stronger, healthier, and more radiant. You know that processed, unhealthy junk foods drain you of your energy and leave you feeling sluggish and moody. You now eat foods that are your life force, filling your body with the nutrients you need to be vibrant and healthy. You see yourself getting healthier, with a more radiant glow.

### #4 Get Physically Active

Imagine that you love getting physically active and taking care of your body. Picture yourself in your ideal body, which is toned, fit, strong, and lean. Imagine you love the feeling of being active and enjoying your fit, energetic body. Now imagine you are walking, going to yoga or Zumba class, excited about caring for your body. Imagine that "moving" is powerful, creating a high level of energy in your body. As you start to exercise, expect your energy levels to improve first, and then over time, you will begin to activate and strengthen your muscles. You actually want to keep walking, running, and moving because you have strength and endurance in your perfect ideal body.

Your bones, muscles, tissues, and cells all vibrate with energy as the weight just melts off your body. You end your workout feeling refreshed, energized, and strong. You know your weight-loss goals will be achievable because you love to take care of your body. You now have all the energy you need to have an amazing day at work.

### #5 Heal Your Body

Imagine every cell in your body filling with healing light. Every part of your body is filled with healing powers so that you feel no aches and pains at all. Your bones, arms, legs, face, and back glow with healing powers. Your heart is filled with healing love and glows brightly. The blood flows through your body, bringing healing to different parts of your body. As the blood flows, it removes any blockages or diseases that you have. Anything that is not functioning properly in the body is instantly healed. All of your energy channels in your body are unblocked and flowing easily. Any bad bacteria, yeasts, and parasites die and vanish away. All the negative things in the body are cleared out, not causing any symptoms or pain. Your body is full of vitality and is functioning very well.

Your energy channels are flowing all day long. You imagine yourself in your perfect, healthy body with endless energy at work. You have enough energy to be productive at work and enjoy your family at home. You look good, feel good, and are having fun. You are healthy, successful, and glowing because of radiant energy flowing through your body. Everyone you encounter feels the enormous energy radiating from your body. People want to talk to you, hang out with you, and just be in your presence. They feel the healing energy from your body and want to be healed as well. You are a beautiful picture of health, in a cleansed, pure mind and body, residing in your ideal shape.

### #6 Create Tight, Elastic, Radiant Skin

Imagine excess skin from your weight loss being removed from your body. All excess skin is pulled away into the whirlpool and eliminated from your body. Your skin is tight and toned all over your body and you cannot even pinch any excess skin because there is none. You feel your skin getting tighter and tighter and all excess fat melting away from your body. By eating healthy, natural, organic foods, you keep your insides clean and begin to look radiant despite your age.

You see yourself walking on the beach and your body is tight and toned. You feel like you have the perfect, ideal body for you. Each day, month after month, you see the excess skin melting away and your body getting more toned and firm. Your excess skin is constantly being pulled into the whirlpool and your whole body is glowing. You are fit, healthy, strong, tight, and toned and you easily maintain your ideal body shape.

### #7 Create A Loving, Supportive Environment

Imagine you have protection and you are safe and secure with tons of love and support all around you. Every ounce of your being feels loves and supported. When you feel off track, you have people in your life to keep you encouraged, motivated, and focused. You have extra support and encouragement when life gets hectic and stressful. You do not easily break promises to yourself because you have a strong support system encouraging you every day. You are able to remain accountable to healthy living due to your support system.

Imagine that in your home there are people who make you feel safe, calm, protected, and nurtured. There is no conflict in your home because of the radiant energy you bring to it. Everyone feels happy, safe, protected, secure, and loving toward you.

### #8 Release Pain, Hurts, and Disappointments

Imagine that every hurt, pain, and disappointment in your life is released from your body. Every hurtful thing that has been stored deep within your cells is released. You let go and wash away all hurt and pain. You let go. You release. You forgive. You move on. You forgive those who have hurt you because forgiveness saves you the trouble of arguing and fighting. It allows you to simply let go. You no longer have to worry about how to punish anyone. You forgive all transgressors and turn them over to God, who can be counted on to deal with them His way.

Forgiveness is really for you, not the other person. It allows you to move on and make your burdens lighter. Forgiveness is the ultimate healing tool that heals your emotional and physical self. It allows you to release the extra weight that you have been carrying in your body. You release any emotional hurt out of the cells of your body, letting them wash away never to return. Every cell in your body can simply let go, and the pain, hurt, and disappointment goes with it. You see people noticing how much lighter and vibrant you are as the weight of your burdens releases from your body.

### #9 Eliminate Food Cravings

Imagine you are offered cake or pie—foods you used to crave daily—and you are no longer tempted by them. You do not have a taste for them anymore. You turn up your nose at these foods because you simply do not want them. You no longer desire or crave junk foods that you used to crave. You do not want any part of those foods and just walk away from them. You see yourself craving healthy, nutrient-rich foods that nourish and sustain your body. These foods are vibrant, fresh, and colorful and your body craves them. These foods keep you energized all day.

The more you eat healthier foods, the more vibrant you become. Unhealthy cravings no longer rule your mind. You are free from food addictions. Everything in life is flowing with positivity and energy.

### #10 Improve Your Digestion

Imagine healing energies throughout your digestive tract from your mouth to your esophagus, through your stomach and your small and large intestines. The healing energies cleanse your digestive tract, cleaning out all toxins, bad bacteria, parasites, and yeast that may be in your gut.

Your entire digestive tract is glowing with healing energies, creating a brand-new digestive system with no impurities or toxins. The digestive tract is healed and regenerated, allowing you to eat without any digestive distress or sluggishness. You eat healthy, live foods. You take probiotics and digestive enzymes to maintain gut health. You have healthy bowel movements with little to no gas or bloating. Eating is so enjoyable, and you truly love your food choices as your body rewards you with its increased energy.

### #11 Reduce Stress

Imagine yourself calm, centered, and confident in your ideal body shape. Now think about what the rest of your day is going to be like. Do you work in an office, school, warehouse? Do you work from home? Imagine your day flowing smoothly, easily, without much drama and stress. Fill your body with a calm and relaxed energy that radiates throughout your day.

As people walk up to you at work, imagine solving their problems and being productive. Whatever work challenges you face, you find creative solutions and bring value to your work environment. No work issues bother you because you are confident, relaxed, and qualified. You radiate positivity and find creative solutions for all situations. You are under control and knowledgeable in meetings, and people listen to what you have to say. Folks want to be around you and do business with you because of your cool, calm, collected demeanor. You have so much energy, and your workday goes by so fast. You enjoy a healthy lunch and appreciate your nutritious foods, eating them slowly and deliberately.

At the end of the day, you leave work feeling calm and relaxed because it was another successful day. You go home to a loving environment where you enjoy your family and friends. Work leaves you feeling energized and wonderful because the day was so successful. You now have enough energy to go work out, take a walk, or play with your kids. You have all the energy you need to enjoy your family and friends. You go to bed looking forward to the next work day because you know every single work day will bring new challenges and opportunities that you are fully equipped to solve. You will win at work each and every day.

### #12 Create Abundance in Your Life

Imagine you have a life filled with loving relationships and financial prosperity, overflowing with abundance. Imagine you have more professional success than you could have ever believed possible in your lifetime. Imagine you are overflowing with love, happiness, success, wealth, health, prosperity, and fitness. Imagine all these things happening in your life.

Imagine you have allowed greatness into every aspect of your life. Imagine you have become great and every cell in your body embodies greatness. You live a life of passion and success because you live up to your true potential. Day after day, you see life becoming healthier, happier, and more successful. You continue to watch the weight melting off and you see yourself living in your ideal body. You are living a life of purpose and you see your purpose manifested in the world. You manifest greatness and live your full potential in every aspect of life. You continue to grow and expand your knowledge and gifts. You remain on a mission and continue to fulfill your purpose.

Imagine you have mastered how to create success in every aspect of your life—spiritual, emotional, physical, financial, and professional. Your success is so overflowing that it floods out of your body and into the world. Your relationships at home and at work are loving and supportive. Your friendships are fun and rewarding. Your happiness and energy cause people to come up to you and ask for your help in directing them to similar success. They want to change their life because you are so amazingly successful. You are a magnet that draws people to you. They want your help with making decisions for their own life. They want the same energetic, healthy, happy life that you live. You know that for the rest of your life, you will be overflowing with abundance and be wildly successful in every aspect of your life.

## CONCLUSION

I hope you have the same success that so many others have had using visualization to achieve dramatic weight loss. You too can become slimmer and healthier and end the struggle with weight forever. Commit to doing visualization for a few minutes each day to reap its tremendous benefits.

# 8

# Commit to Losing Weight

I LOVE SPORTS AND so does the rest of my family. My youngest brother probably is the biggest sports fan in the family. When he was a toddler, he preferred to watch sports on television to Saturday-morning cartoons. If our mother changed the channel from a football game to cartoons, he would have a fit! One day when my brother was older, I asked him if he had a favorite sport. He responded, "I'm interested in all sports, but I'm committed to basketball." I said to him, "You're *committed* to basketball? What does that even mean?" He said something I had not really thought about. His answer made me realize that *not everything we are interested in is something we are truly committed to*.

My brother explained that he is interested in sports because they are fun, challenging, and emotional. There is a sense of pride and a feeling of accomplishment watching your hometown team win. He is also competitive, and sports bring about the purest form of competition: there is a winner and there is a loser. It does not get much more black and white than that.

However, with basketball the feelings go deeper. My brother is *motivated* by basketball. When he is playing basketball, he is motivated to practice harder to be the best player he can be. Or, if he is watching his favorite teams, he will cheer them on with pronounced passion because he craves the sensation of winning. My brother told me that there is a level of self-control and discipline attributed to just about anything basketball-related that is unmatched in other sports or pursuits of interest. When his coach implored him to shoot extra jump shots after practice, he didn't complain. He knew those extra shots would make him a better player, and he was committed to being a better player. My brother did not have the same level of motivation or discipline in other sports as he did for basketball. He likes football, baseball, and other sports, but only basketball can push him to work his hardest and elicit the kind of discipline necessary to make sacrifices needed to achieve his desired results. When it comes to all things basketball, my brother is committed to doing whatever it takes to enjoy the sport to the fullest and be the best at it.

What about you? Are you committed to losing weight or are you just interested? For my brother, commitment was a little easier because of his love for basketball. Losing weight and keeping it off permanently is hard and can seem like an impossible task. I do not know many people who love hard work and seemingly impossible tasks. You may love the feeling of how you look after you have lost weight but enjoying the actual process? That is a rarity (or at least from my experience it is). For this reason, committing to losing weight and keeping it off permanently is going to take motivation, discipline, and willpower.

In this chapter, we will cover the different forms of motivation that influence our behaviors. It is important to understand the different types of motivation to determine which inspires us the most to lose weight and keep it off. We will also learn how to maintain the willpower and discipline necessary to stay the course until we have achieved the weight-loss goals we set for ourselves.

However, before we can start exploring different types of motivation that best light a fire to keep us along our weight-loss journey, we first must make sure we are not merely interested but actually *committed* to this process. To do so, let us define the characteristics of a truly committed person.

## INTERESTED VS. COMMITTED

It is great to be someone who has multiple interests in a variety of topics. Often the most gregarious people you meet have interests in a wide range of subjects. It is why interesting people are enjoyable to talk to. They can hold a conversation on something that is dear to you and you will feel like they understand. People with multiple interests are good listeners because they enjoy learning something new, a new curiosity to pique their interest. Our sociable friends can use what they have learned from you in other social settings to strike up conversations and engage folks in an effort to share the knowledge or simply make conversation to pass the time. The more things they know (at least on a surface level), the more things they have to talk about to engage people. There is also a quality of being a good listener that should not get overlooked either. Think about it, it is hard to expand your interest barometer if you do not listen and find an appreciation in what others are telling you. For example, let us say you and I are having a conversation about music and I start to talk to you about my favorite type of music—hip-hop. As soon as I start to go into detail about why I prefer this particular genre, you tune me out. How is that beneficial to our conversation? Communication is a two-way street. Our conversation will die if you talk and do not hear a word I say.

Interested people are sociable, outgoing, and good listeners. They are willing to talk to just about anyone and listen to almost everything people have to say. Personally, I *like* interested people, but I *love* committed people. Interested people are numerous and commonplace. Put me in a social gathering and I can spot the interested ones immediately.

Committed people, however, are fewer in number and harder to find. Committed people tend to break away from the group when they notice others around them do not have the same drive toward results. A committed person moves with precision and operates as if they have a plan and everything they do is in support of that plan. *For committed people, there are no excuses, only results.* It is a desire for accomplishment that separates them from the pack. However, having desire is not all it takes; in fact, it is just the start. Your desire is what helps you separate things you are only interested in from the ones you are willing to put real effort into. However, you have to then decide to act and put in the work necessary to fulfill your desires.

As for my brother and his love of basketball, here is another quick story of how his desire pushed him to reach his goal. My brother was committed to earning a starting spot on the varsity basketball team. He knew he was a great passer and a great defender and adept at attacking the rim. However, he had a desire to be great, not just good, and he would not be considered great (at least in his coach's eyes) until he improved his jump shot. To get to starter level, he decided to go all in and commit to becoming a better jump shooter. The level of commitment my brother made was to shoot hundreds and hundreds of jump shots every day over the summer to the point where he became a lights-out shooter. When practice opened up that next fall, the coach noticed his improved jump shot and, before the first scrimmage, he made my brother a starter. My brother accomplished his goal as varsity starter because he decided nothing under his control would hold him back. When you are committed to something, you accept zero excuses. You accept only results!

My brother loves basketball above all the other sports and is committed. He had a desire to become a better player and decided he was going to do what was required to get to the level he set as his goal—being a starter on the varsity team. That is what we must do to reach our weight-loss goals: separate what we are only interested in from what we are truly committed to, establish a desire to be better, and decide to put in the necessary work to achieve our weight-loss goals.

*Making sacrifices and putting in the necessary work is commitment.* People fail in trying to lose weight not because of a lack of interest but because of a failure to commit. How do we avoid failure and find the desire to make the sacrifices necessary to lose weight and feel better about ourselves? It starts with motivation. You must find the motivation necessary to keep yourself on track and commit to putting in the work every single day until you have reached the point where goals and milestones are being met.

Here are some tips for moving from Interested in Losing Weight to Committed to Losing Weight:

1. *Write Down Your Commitment:* A common success factor for weight loss is putting your commitment in writing, as this will increase your chance of success. Think of your commitment as a promise that you are making to yourself. By writing it down, you can refer to it later and it will help you continue making progress.

2. *Tell Your Close Circle (Family and Friends):* Do not try to go it alone. Seek the support of family and friends so they can help keep you accountable to your weight-loss goals. Having a good support system can make all the difference in staying truly committed to your success.

3. *Get Your Mind Right:* Adjust your mind-set in terms of what you say and think. Success begins in the mind so use the seven mental strategies in this book to build the mental mastery necessary to achieve your weight-loss goals. You will have to create a permanent shift in thoughts, feelings, habits, and behaviors about weight loss in order to have long-term success.

4. *Plan for Success:* Just saying you want to lose weight is not a plan. If you were to decide to get a new job, you would update your résumé, use online job searches, and schedule and prepare for interviews. You would plan to achieve your goal of finding a new job. The

same goes for weight loss. It requires a plan of what weight-loss system you will follow, going grocery shopping, getting a support system, an exercise routine, et cetera. Take time to plan your weight loss for the greatest success.

5. *Set a Deadline:* Set a time frame for when you want to reach your first weight-loss goal. A goal without a deadline is less likely to be achieved. Set a deadline, create a plan, and work your plan.

In the next section, we will take a look at the different types of motivation that help to influence our behaviors and identify the types of motivation that best suit each personality.

## COMMITMENT AND MOTIVATION

Studies have shown different forms of motivation influence our behavior in their own unique ways. What we need to do is tap into those motivations that most effectively influence our behaviors and actions toward losing weight and keeping it off. There are four common forms of motivation: *incentive, fear, achievement,* and *social.* Let us take a closer look and define each relative to losing weight.

### Incentive

Incentive is a form of motivation that revolves around the idea of rewards. The rewards can be monetary or nonmonetary in nature. The key that defines this type of motivation is a desire to do something based upon the idea at the end or when the action is completed, you will be recompensed. If you are the type of person who likes to be compensated for your efforts, or simply enjoys the reward itself, then this type of motivation is ideal for you.

To take advantage of this form of motivation to help you achieve your weight goals, set incremental goals or milestones. At the end of each one, reward yourself for achieving the goal. The thought here is that by setting multiple milestones, you are giving yourself multiple opportunities to be rewarded. I recommend reaching out to the people in your support system and allowing them to be in charge of doling out the rewards. The rewards should vary and be equivalent to the level of effort required to reach the goal. In other words, if the achievement is minor or an entry-level type of accomplishment, then the reward should be small. I will not define what is considered major or minor in terms of goals because we are all at different stages in our weight-loss journey and in this context, goals are relative. However, use common sense. Do not reward yourself with a week of cheat days after hitting the very first goal.

## Fear

The next form of motivation, fear, involves consequences. Motivation through fear is the antithesis of motivation through incentive. When motivation through incentive fails, fear is the next best alternative. A common expression when discussing motivation is "the carrot and the stick." The carrot represents an incentive while the stick represents fear. What are your fears when it comes to losing weight and eating healthy? Write them down, make a mental note. Acknowledging your fears is the first step toward turning them into a positive motivator. If your fear is not being a certain size when you walk down the aisle of your own wedding, or of dying before you see your grandkids grow up, or of being dissatisfied with the reflection you see in the mirror, then whenever you're feeling discouraged about losing weight, reflect on the trepidation these feelings caused. Turn your fear into a positive force and use it as willpower to propel you toward your goals.

We have to be careful when using fear as a motivator, however. If you are the type of person who does not perform well under pressure or if you are anxious to a fault, then fear may not be the best type of motivation for you. The last thing we want is for your fears to inundate you and impede your progress. I recommend acknowledging the worst of your fears when it comes to losing weight. If simply the thought of these fears leaves you frozen and completely overwhelmed, stop and reset your mind to positive thoughts. Try another type of motivation.

### Achievement

If you are on this journey to lose weight, eat clean, and live a healthy lifestyle, then naturally you have a desire for self-improvement. This is why you have set goals for yourself: the goals measure your performance. When thinking of motivation in terms of achievement, we refer to our drive for competency. We are driven by our goals and desire to improve to affirm competency in ourselves and to others. Whether your stated goal is to lose 20 pounds, 50 pounds, or even 100 pounds, achieving your goal is your chance to show others you can accomplish what you set out to do. It is your opportunity to show others and, perhaps most important, yourself, that you are competent.

While others may be happy, you accomplished whatever goals you set for yourself, no one will likely feel more satisfied than you will. After all, you put in the hard work, made the sacrifices, and pushed through when things looked bleak. You were motivated to achieve your goal, prove you were competent so you deserve self-congratulation! A little external recognition is welcome too. Whether it be a lofty reward or a simple pat on the back, acknowledgment from others can go a long way in helping to keep you motivated toward your goals. When relying on motivation via achievement, it does not matter if praise of accomplishment comes from internal satisfaction or recognition of others as long the drive for competency is met.

### Social

Social motivation is the desire to belong or be accepted by your peers. Social motivation is highly influential in the drive to lose weight. It feels good to be complimented and received favorably by your peers. However, be cautious about relying too much on the approval of others. No matter how much weight you may have lost or how great you look, there will always be someone to bring you down. I do not know why some people feel the need to talk badly about others or be discouraging. Perhaps it is a way for them to feel good about themselves. Regardless, you do not need to worry or focus any attention on people like this at all. They are roadblocks in your journey to be avoided, ignored, and dismissed outright!

When drawing upon social motivation to push you toward

your goals, look to your support group, family, friends, and people you trust. These are the people who have your best interests at heart and whose opinions you should value. When you look good, they will be the ones to tell you. When there is still a little more work to do to get you to your best self, they will be sure to politely tell you so as well. It is totally cool and even valuable to be motivated by the affection of your loved ones, just make sure it is the right group of supportive people whose opinions you heed.

Each type of motivation has its positives and negatives. Basing it upon your personality type, you should know which will be most effective in helping you stay committed to your goal of losing weight and eating healthy. These four motivating types—incentive, fear, achievement, and social—are presented as a guide to help you understand the types of common drivers people use in everyday life. It is not to say one is better than the other or even have you focus solely on one motivation factor. Feel free to use them all if they are applicable to your situation. There is a time to push yourself using fear, or to feel inspired with a little incentive, or to simply strive for the recognition of your peers. The key is that you use whatever motivation strategy is most effective at the most opportune time to light a fire under your butt to stay committed to your goal of losing weight and keeping it off.

## CONCLUSION

Commitment is essential to losing weight and keeping it off, which is a long-term investment in yourself to get better each and every day. Start by setting a goal. In the beginning, you are going to need plenty of willpower to push through the tough times. Multiple goals may put too many unnecessary demands on your mind and body in the beginning stages. Focus on one goal, and use your motivation and willpower to help you accomplish that goal. Accomplishing goals is major and deserves praise. Can you stay motivated and committed to losing weight and living healthy? Or are you simply just interested in losing weight?

# 9

---

# Control Your Emotions

---

JUST THE THOUGHT of some foods make us feel comfortable, safe, and warm. Comfort foods take us to a comfortable time or place in our life. For me, my aunt's sweet potato pie reminds of me of love and family.

Comfort foods are not all bad. Occasionally eating comfort foods can be part of a healthy relationship with food. However, if food becomes the first thing you think about when you are feeling sad, hurt, or lonely, then food has become a destructive coping mechanism. Some overweight people are using food like a drug to numb the pain and often end up in a food coma. They use food to sedate themselves the same way alcoholics use alcohol to avoid experiencing pain or feelings of sadness or loneliness. This can often cause them to be detached from life, friends, and family. It can get so bad that they become depressed and do not even want to go to work. The struggle with emotional eating is one of the primary reasons folks cannot maintain a healthy weight. However, you can end your struggle with emotional eating once and for all.

## BEWARE OF EMOTIONAL EATING

Do you eat when you are sad, hurt, or lonely? Emotional eating almost always leads to inappropriate eating. Without realizing it, you may be caught in a vicious cycle of "living to eat," not "eating to live." Just the same as a drug or alcohol addict, you have to make sure that you do not use food to escape your problems. See food for what it is: fuel for the body to give it energy and vitality.

An important way to address emotional eating is to learn the difference between emotional hunger and physical hunger. This is absolutely key. Sometimes our relationship with food is an emotional one rather than a physical one. Sometimes we eat to fill an emotional gap or some other negative emotion. But no food—be it a cracker, a piece of cake, a scoop of ice cream, or a slice of pie—can satisfy emotional hunger.

Physical hunger comes about gradually about every three to four hours. Emotional hunger comes on suddenly—I must eat something now. But you rarely feel satisfied or full, and so you just keep eating and eating until the entire bag of chips or pint of ice cream is gone. If the hunger comes on after an argument or a negative emotion, then it is emotional hunger. Rather than deal with the emotions head on, you turn to food. Watch the clock. If you ate a meal and were full one hour ago and then feel a sudden need to eat something, it is probably emotional hunger.

Dealing with your emotional issues will help you improve

your relationship with food. To deal with your emotions, you must come to understand that the bad things that have happened in your life have probably been floating around in your mind for years, and because you try to suppress these feelings, as most of us do, they have never been properly processed.

When we dwell on the sad events of our lives, they get etched in our minds, stuck in our bodies, weighing us down emotionally. We must process these experiences and let them go. If we do not, the negative emotions become toxic to our emotional and physical body. Sad or painful experiences need to be processed, they are not meant to linger for years and years.

Just as we can get rid of toxic wastes in the body, we can get rid of toxic emotions. Instead of eating to distract ourselves from bad feelings, we need to process and eliminate them, just like the body does with food: it takes the nutrients it needs and expels the rest.

## EMBRACE YOUR FEELINGS

Many of us have not mastered how to feel our feelings. However, when we do not process our emotions, they are often displaced onto the body and stored in the flesh as fat. The only way to remove the weight of unprocessed emotions is to allow ourselves to feel them. Just as food needs to be chewed and digested in the stomach, emotions need to be felt and processed in the mind. For emotional eaters, as soon as the emotion hits, they turn to food to avoid feeling those emotions.

Emotions are there to tell you something. They carry messages. Emotions need to be felt, acknowledged, and processed. Do not be quick to suppress or ignore them—or worse, eat to avoid feeling them. Maybe you grew up in a house where your parent said, "Stop crying or I'll give you something to cry about." So you learned to suppress your feelings instead of crying and feeling them. At a very young age, you learned to not really experience your own feelings. If the feelings were traumatic or violent, you learned to numb the pain as a coping mechanism.

We think by suppressing our feelings, they will go away, but they don't, they just go somewhere else, namely into the form of excess weight on the body. Think of your cravings for unhealthy foods as an emotional outcry or temper tantrum. You can choose to feel the emotion, honor it, and process it so the miraculous transformation can happen in your body and the weight can be released, or you can choose to suppress the feeling and cause it to be stored in your physical body as excess weight. You always have a choice. Spiritual mastery comes from surrendering to your higher self, not trying to handle everything in your mortal mind/body.

Surrendering these feelings will release them from you. Let's say you went through a painful divorce, your spouse passed away, or you were beaten violently—you will experience grief and pain. But that is not where the story ends. These feelings can be felt and processed in your life. You will emerge stronger and wiser, but only after you have felt the pain. You will learn to love again after a broken heart. Avoiding the pain makes you weaker. Feeling the pain makes you stronger. If you wake up sad, it only means you are a human being with emotions. Regardless of your feelings, there is no reason to run from them or use food to escape from them. Your feelings are always there to teach you something or to help you grow spiritually.

To heal your spiritual self, first feel the emotion and whatever pain is associated with it. Over time, the emotion will no longer have power over you. You will no longer experience suffering from it. It is released and no longer pushed into your flesh, allowing the excess weight to be released as well.

## WHY DO PEOPLE STRUGGLE WITH EMOTIONAL EATING?

Oftentimes people think that they are overeating because the food tastes good, but in reality, it goes much deeper than that. And it is not only that you may be dealing with deep-seated emotional issues. Rather than just getting through, life's stress and hassles can trigger you to overeat and grab unhealthy junk foods to make life easier.

Let's consider the most common reasons people struggle with emotional eating.

### Boredom

The most common reason people overeat is out of boredom. When you are bored, the experience of eating food breaks the monotony. It typically happens when you are watching nonstimulating television programs, enjoying a lazy Sunday, studying for an exam, killing time, or are just bored at work. If you are the type that always has to stay busy, anytime you have some downtime, you eat because you just have to be doing something. You have to fill any hole in your schedule with eating. Understanding boredom will help put an end to this emotional trigger that causes overeating.

### Frustration and Anger

If you overindulge in eating a lot of crunchy foods, like chips and cookies, it is believed that you are frustrated or angry. The physical act of biting and crunching serves as a way to release feelings of anger and frustration. Some people eat ice or hard candy to release feelings of anger as well. The next time you reach for crunchy foods, stop to think if you are frustrated or angry.

### Reward

Have you ever rewarded yourself with food for finishing a chore, such as studying or cleaning the house? Eating can be a motivation to accomplish some undesirable task. We do this with children all the time—for instance, offer to give them ice cream or cookies as a reward if they behave. Even at the gym, people will reward themselves with a muffin or croissant if they have a good workout. Using food as a reward helps us get through challenging or mundane tasks because it makes them tolerable if we know we have food as our reward.

### Lack of Excitement

When life becomes dull, we often use the eating experience as a way to add excitement. A dinner reservation at a favorite restaurant, for example, is exciting. You just cannot wait to get there. Also, when you first start a diet, you are so full of hope, but when you fall off the diet, you feel down. Then you overindulge in unhealthy foods to try to recreate the excitement and hope again. So we diet and overeat, diet and overeat repeatedly. Some folks have dealt with so much pain and hurt that they eat sweets to counter the bitterness they feel each day. Just trying to bring sweetness into their life.

## Food as a Display of Love

Food can be a reflection of love. Relatives, especially mothers, often show us love through some food that they have prepared for us. For some, even if love was lacking at home, there was always plenty of food to eat. When you are in a new romantic relationship and your partner serves you a home-cooked meal, that typically means the relationship is moving to a higher level. Food has always been used as a signifier of love and caring.

## Stress

Many people eat to cope with stress. Some people experience stressful situations all throughout the day, every day, and this can lead to excessive fat, particularly belly fat. When you are stressed, your body releases cortisol (also known as the stress hormone). Fat caused by stress (i.e., stress fat) stores in the belly. Studies have shown that when cortisol is released into the bloodstream, you become less sensitive to leptin, the hormone that tells your brain you are full. When this happens, you tend to eat more and begin to crave sugar. That means that your body not only slows down your metabolism when you are stressed out, it actually tells you to consume more food.

## *Mild Depression*

It is very common for folks to turn to food if they are feeling depressed. When people are experiencing mild depression, they also experience weight gain. They interpret their feelings as hunger and they eat to soothe their feelings.

## HOW TO HANDLE EMOTIONAL EATING

You will first have to face the feelings that are eating at you day in and day out. Acknowledge what is troubling you and allow these feelings to come to the forefront so you do not have to push them down with food.

Here are some suggestions for how to deal with your feelings:

- Write your feelings in a diary journal.
- Call a trusted friend or relative and talk through your feelings.
- Talk with a psychologist or therapist.
- Confront the person who is the root cause of your toxic feelings.
- Cry it out.
- Find a hobby that you truly enjoy.
- Read a good book or watch a movie.
- Take a nap and rest.

## DEALING WITH CHALLENGING OR STRESSFUL SITUATIONS

So what do you do when you are in the middle of a challenging or stressful situation and your best intentions fall through? We have the best intentions, but we get challenged trying to process our emotions and give in to unhealthy eating. One thing I have come to realize is that we can only do our best and make peace with ourselves when we fall off track. I always say, it is about progress, not perfection.

You will need to have practical strategies that help you get through those tough times more easily so you can avoid falling off track.

### *Celebrations*

Celebrations are a frequent and important part of everyone's life. It is the time to express love and appreciation to someone during holidays, birthdays, weddings, and many other events. It is the time to bond with family and friends and simply enjoy the fellowship and company of others. So much of advertising and marketing centers around celebrations, particularly around wine, liquor, and beer. It is as if they use celebrations as a reason to market and sell junk food. Even in the grocery store, they use every opportunity to encourage you to indulge yourself when celebrating this holiday or that holiday. Now, of course, if you want to celebrate with others and make it a special occasion, that is perfectly fine, but be sure to focus on the fellowship with others—on enjoying quality time with loved ones. In reality, eating is not the problem. God gave us food for nourishment, satisfaction, and even celebration. The problem is when food becomes too big a part of our total pleasure in life.

If you want to attend the celebration but not indulge in unhealthy foods, do not feel emotionally pressured to eat what you feel is bad for you. You do not have to eat high-sugar, high-fat foods to please other people. I know that can be hard, but there are strategies that will help you avoid the pressure. Even if you are having a great time socializing, you do not have to give in to peer pressure. Feel free to take a walk or call a support buddy or find some excuse to get away from the gathering for a while. Enjoy yourself, let go of your eating restrictions, or resist any foods that cause you to fall off track. You are in control.

## TIPS FOR DEALING WITH CHALLENGING OR STRESSFUL SITUATIONS

Here are some common pitfalls and solutions for those who lose control and fall off track.

### Have an Escape Plan

If you feel pressured or uncomfortable at a family gathering, have a plan for leaving or at least for taking a break. Go to another room, run errands to the grocery store, or pick up an elderly relative. Also, it may be best to drive your own car so you come and go when it is convenient for you. If your friends or loved ones are upsetting you, you do not want to be stuck waiting for your ride to leave. Always be prepared to leave when it is best for you.

## Start New Traditions

You can also start a new tradition and bring the one healthy meal to the celebration. But it should not be just a healthy meal but an outstanding meal that shocks everyone when they find out that it is clean and healthy. In my book *Green Smoothies for Life*, we have dozens of outstanding meals that will impress. You could be the relative known for bringing something special and nontraditional that they will love as it's also good for the body. As an example, I used to bring gluten-free, sugar-free brownies with walnuts that everyone loved. Folks were so glad to know they could indulge without feeling guilty.

## Create Laughter and Love

Many times when family gets together, they bring up old, painful memories and emotional subjects. I remember one time at Thanksgiving, two relatives got into an argument and one of them flipped over the Thanksgiving table with all the good food on it. It was devastating not to have all that delicious food that took hours to cook.

Sometimes relatives create so much drama that watching it is like theater. Like a movie or Broadway show, it can certainly be entertaining, but do not let it consume you. Sometimes just let it play out, watch, and just stay out of it. Enjoy the craziness in other people as some have been that way for life and are not really going to change. See the humor in the situation. Humor is powerful because it is based upon truth. Truth can make people feel embarrassed, anxious, or hurt but as the saying goes: the truth can set you free. Take the awkwardness away by laughing to yourself. Sure, some family members will not like you making light of some heavy topic because they thrive on conflict and negativity and want everyone to live in that place. You do not have to, you can laugh to yourself and keep it moving.

## Manage through Loss and Grief

Holiday gathering and family celebrations often remind us of loved ones we have lost. When a loss is fresh, it can definitely bring up lots of pain and sadness. Even before the gathering, you may begin to feel irritable and sad as you feel the loss of a loved one again. Loss can include a marriage or relationship that has ended. If you spent holidays with your spouse or significant other and the marriage dissolved, holidays can remind you of the love lost or the dream marriage that did not last forever. If you had special holiday traditions, it will be important to create new ones so that the holidays remind you of happier times and happier memories.

Do not drown yourself in sadness and get depressed during the holidays. Feel the sadness and hurt and then move on to happier times in your life. I lost my dad over twenty-five years ago, and holidays still remind me of him. Even though it has been a very long time, I remember the last Christmas we spent together because he said, "Let's enjoy this one because this will likely be the last Christmas we spend together as a family." I will never forget those words and how painful they were. He was right. However, I have learned to enjoy Christmas celebrations with family members, while still cherishing the last Christmas with my dad.

Think about the times of the year when you experienced significant loss. Do you notice that those times you are more emotional, irritable, and moody? Write in a journal about your feelings and your experiences so you do not experience emotional overload during those times. This will help you to be prepared to nurture yourself so that you can minimize the impact on you. Deliberately do things that lift your spirits, like traveling, volunteering at your church, Christmas caroling, or going to the movies. Whatever it takes to cope and heal, do that and allow yourself to feel better.

### Love Yourself through Sickness

Sometimes too much stress and drama in your life can lower your immune system and cause you to get sick. Being sick can be stressful in and of itself and make you upset or anxious, causing you to stay sick for long periods of time. For many, they want to feed a cold or just eat a lot of comfort foods to feel better. When you are sick, however, that is the most important time to eat healthy and get enough sleep to allow your body to recover and to boost its immune system. Eating unhealthy slows the recovery process time.

When you are achy, tired, or irritable, stay hydrated, eat healthy, rest, and drink plenty of liquids to help your body flush out toxins. If you work out a lot, this may be a time to take a few days off from strenuous workouts so that you do not put too much stress on your body. Doing light exercises like nonstrenuous yoga (Vinyasa, Bikram, Ashtanga), walking, or stretching may be best for a speedy recovery. This is not the time to obsess over your weight and stress about missing workouts.

### *Don't Lose Your Mind on Vacations and Work Travel*

So many people ask how to stay on track while traveling for work or while on vacation. I always say we have to do a bit more planning, but every restaurant on the road has healthy options. You can also bring or simply purchase healthy snacks while traveling. It is simply not true that you cannot stay on track on vacations or work travel.

A little bit of planning goes a long way. You can figure out in advance what restaurants have healthier foods or where the healthy grocery stores are near your hotel. There are a few things I always have on me when I travel, such as nuts and seeds, protein bars, and popcorn. These snacks always hold me over and help me stay on track. Even airports have food kiosks with fruits, veggies, hummus, and other healthy snacks. You can be successful while traveling, it is just about proper planning and a decision to choose healthy.

### *Manage Moods through Hormonal Imbalances*

For women, especially those over thirty-five years old, hormonal shifts make it difficult to maintain stable moods and emotions. For many, mood changes start during PMS. For others, they may occur during perimenopause/menopause. But most women have mood shifts at some point in their life. Men too can experience mood change due to hormonal shifts. Both men and women can experience emotional instability and even depression.

In addition to mood changes, men and women can experience sudden weight gain due to hormonal shifts as they age, which contributes to them feeling emotionally overwhelmed in their forties, fifties, and sixties. If you often feel angry, sad, sensitive, and moody, know that it is time to get your hormones tested. Hormones affect how you feel, how you look, and, most important, how you maintain your weight and health. When your hormones are balanced properly, you will have great health, beauty, and vibrancy. When your hormones are imbalanced, you have mood swings, you crave unhealthy foods, and you feel sluggish and lethargic.

I once had an unexplained weight gain of thirty pounds, practically overnight, in just a few months. However, after balancing my hormones, I was able to feel emotionally stable and get back to my ideal weight. You too can achieve hormonal balance and know that when your hormones are functioning at their optimal levels, your body is at its peak performance and maintains your healthy, ideal weight.

### Develop a Healthy Relationship with Food

The eating habits of an overweight person are often impulsive, driven by fear, and out of control. The solution to overeating is not to starve yourself and deny yourself food altogether. You do not have to be fearful of food or scared to eat anything.

The only way to attain a healthy relationship with food is to learn to love it and ensure that the food you put into your body loves you back: it fuels you, nourishes you, and supports your optimal health and vitality. A candy bar does not love you—it is full of sugar and processed chemicals that harm your body. The people who made it do not love you either—they are just trying to make money by selling you a product. Chemicals and processed foods lead to poor health, sickness, food allergies, ailments, and other diseases, none of which I would classify as "loving" conditions. If you are in a place where you still desire candy, that just means that you are still growing spiritually and learning healthier eating habits.

Foods that love you are those that contribute to your health and wellness, such as fruits, nuts and seeds, and vegetables. These healthy, natural foods make your body stronger and able to fight illness and disease, and have beauty and vibrancy. Natural, healthy foods make your body strong, fight illness, restore your body, produce beautiful skin, revitalize your mind, give you energy, slow the aging process, and will taste so much better than you can imagine once your taste buds have been reprogrammed. You have to be deliberate about finding healthy foods because unhealthy foods are readily available and easily accessible. But in some instances, I bet you have driven right by the farmers' market or health food store. It is time to make a stop there and begin to change your life.

Do not stress about trying to stop eating unhealthy foods at the beginning of your journey. It is a process that involves breaking your addictions to the many unhealthy foods you eat and think you "love" today. Just be aware of exactly what you are eating and know that there will come a day when you will no longer love foods that do not love you.

For me, I overcame my addiction to sugar, sweets, and junk food over time by taking gradual steps. Instead of eating regular chocolate chip cookies with refined white sugar, I began to eat sugar-free cookies that contained artificial sweeteners. Although they were not very healthy, due to either the white flour, trans fats, and artificial sweeteners they contained, they did help me break my addiction to white refined sugar. Breaking my addiction of white refined sugar was my personal gradual first step. As I continued my journey to eating healthier, I learned about the dangers of artificial sweeteners and trans fats, and that discovery motivated me to stop eating sugar-free cookies as well. You will find the right approach for how you transition to more healthy foods that is right for you and it's going to be gradual.

## CONCLUSION

Some people struggle with their overall weight and food in general. They feel they lack willpower or they are lazy and un-motivated when it comes to eating and exercise. People often make excuses for their excess weight by saying, everyone in my family is overweight so it is hereditary. They also say they do not have enough time to exercise and eat right ever since they in-jured their back, and so they gained a lot of weight. Even though these things, genetic factors, injuries and the like, play a factor in overeating, they are still just excuses that prevent peo-ple from resolving their weight issues.

We all have the ability to maintain a healthy body weight, and it should be a lot easier than it seems at times. Enjoying great food with family and friends enhances our social experi-ences. There is nothing wrong with occasionally enjoying food and celebrating life. The issue is when you use food to cope with the hard times and struggles in life. We have abused food so much that our health and life are at risk. We can make ex-cuses for why we overeat all day, but in the end, the truth is emotional eating represents an inability to love and care for ourselves.

If you struggle with emotional eating, you are not properly connecting to yourself (mind, body, and spirit). When we are truly connected and aligned with our body, mind, and spirit, we know how to meet our physical needs, as well as spiritual and emotional needs. We know what true physical hunger feels like versus emotional hunger. We also know how to process emotions such as sadness, fear, and anger. We have stopped using food to soothe, comfort, calm, and distract us from unpleasant emotions and feelings. You may have stopped asking others for what you need, but you can learn the skills necessary to care for your own needs and put an end to emotional eating.

# 10

## Establish Success Habits

Y OU CANNOT SOLELY rely on willpower and self-control to
lose weight—you have to control your environment and
circumstances. Your ability to maintain self-control will depend on your environment. If your house is hectic and chaotic, or if you are stressed or in a bad mood or easily distracted,
you will struggle to maintain self-control. In order to have
more self-control, you will have to build success into your environment.

When you wake up, what is the first thing you see? What
surrounds you? How have you set up your private space? Your
environment directly impacts the progress you have on your
weight-loss journey. Do you have toxic people in our life? Do
you have unhealthy foods throughout the house? Do you have
mental hazards all over the place? You need to set up your environment properly in order to achieve health and weight-loss

goals. Clear space in your mind, home, and life so that you can avoid setbacks and failures.

Your environment is stronger than your willpower. For example, think about how casinos are designed to influence you while you are there. They have no clocks, no windows, nothing to give you a sense of time or anything to hurry you out of there. The carpet is usually busy with lots of patterns to keep you stimulated and alert. Free drinks are served so you do not have to get up to go buy one. Other environments, such as nightclubs, hotels, and churches, are intentionally designed to bring about a certain kind of behavior as well. Some of these places even consult behavioral psychologists to get the setting just right.

So, ask yourself, how much have you thought about your environment? Do you know if your environment is set up for weight-loss success?

Distractions—like trying to type an email, watch TV, and respond to Facebook posts all at the same time—cause people to struggle on their weight-loss journey. Distractions have become so common throughout our day, and this has been detrimental for dieters. Studies show that dieters eat 40 percent more than nondieters when they are distracted. We do not know why distractions cause dieters to overeat, but studies show that they do.

When folks go to weight-loss boot camps, the entire environment is set up to avoid distractions and anything that may impede success. The "camper" even has doctors to monitor them, trainers to push them, chefs to prepare healthy foods, and everything required to help them achieve success. They have one goal and that is to ensure that you achieve weight-loss success, and everything in the environment is set up to support that goal.

Self-discipline cannot compete with the pure pleasure of eating momma's sweet potato pie. There is a reason that between 90 percent and 95 percent of those who lose weight on a diet regain it all within three years. You are going to need more than self-discipline to win this weight-loss battle.

For too many of us, reliance on self-discipline fails to bring about the change we desire. This is an old model of motivation that said those who can lose weight are disciplined and strong while those who cannot are undisciplined and weak-minded. It is said that self-discipline is something we pull from deep down inside of us, but unfortunately, many of us cannot find it. Studies are showing that self-discipline is playing a very limited role in helping to change one's eating habits. So, we have to ask: How do we create better habits? How long does it take someone to create a habit? *We have to apply effort, not self-discipline.* Self-discipline requires you to change something on the inside (inner world), whereas effort requires you to re-arrange things on the outside (outer world).

When you are in the moment of deciding whether to eat junk or something healthy, self-discipline is often not enough. You probably have experienced that. So instead of self-discipline, you have to focus on effort. Put effort into setting up your outer world (our environment) to allow yourself to succeed. Doing this "pre-handles" the problem before you get tempted to avoid struggling with self-discipline.

You have to control the things in your environment that trigger you to eat unhealthfully or get off track. This is key to long-term success with weight loss. You have to recognize that the human mind is easily tempted. Rather than trying to resist temptation, you are better off rearranging your environment to avoid running into so many temptations.

Let's talk about how this works. How do we rearrange our "outer world" and set up our environment to ensure weight-loss success?

## WHAT ARE SUCCESS HABITS?

A success habit is anything we do or put in our environment for the purpose of helping us avoid temptations throughout the day. This means we prepare things in our physical environment that set us up for weight-loss success. Many of these things are inexpensive and require little effort. Then, over time, success just happens.

I have many success habits in my life now. One, I choose to eat out only in places where I can eat healthy food. My favorite restaurant is one that serves bison steak, sweet potatoes, and green beans. I know I can get a healthy meal at this enjoyable restaurant, so I go there instead of going to an unhealthy Italian restaurant with very few healthy options or a restaurant with buffet. For many, buffets present a particular challenge. The reality is that food is one of the most addictive substances on earth, so we have to have habits in place to avoid overeating.

Another example, liver cleansing has been the most impactful detox method that helps my body burn fat and so I take a liver supplement consistently. You know how I remember to take it every single day? I have the bottle on my nightstand right next to my glasses. I wake up, pick up my glasses, and then take my liver supplement on an empty stomach, with eight ounces of water. This ensures that I consistently take the supplement that has the most positive impact on my weight loss.

My business partner struggled with water intake. He knows how critical water is for weight loss and was determined to find a way to drink more water daily, but somehow, day after day, he never did. He finally installed a water cooler in his office to make it easy to keep a glass of water on his desk. He sees the water cooler and grabs a cup of water as he moves about throughout the day.

We have to acknowledge the deep attachment to food and must respect this so we do not set ourselves up to fail. So, I do not want you to worry about self-discipline. Instead, focus on setting up success habits in your life, which create the habits to help you succeed long-term.

The remainder of this chapter will focus on the most common success habits that people use to avoid temptations and stay on track on their weight-loss journey.

## SUCCESS HABITS TO HELP AVOID TEMPTATIONS

### *1. Prepare your home environment for success.*

Think about what your physical environment looks like. Does it energize you or is it chaotic and hectic? Are there piles of clothes on the floor? Is there one room that you have wanted to clean up? As an example, your bedroom is meant for relaxation and romance: does it create that vibe for you? If not, maybe start there. Start small and just focus on one room that you can organize and clean up so it will make you feel good when you walk into it. See if cleaning and organizing this one room makes you feel energized and lighter on your feet. This will also give you momentum that will allow you to clean and organize the next room. The goal is to clean up small spaces or one room or closet at a time.

### 2. Immerse yourself in learning.

Have you immersed yourself in learning about health and weight loss? If you want to learn and master anything in your life, you have to immerse yourself in it. Let the knowledge consume you. Knowing everything about eating clean and detoxing helped me stay slim. However, unexpected weight gain forced me to learn about my hormones and how they were affecting my weight. I studied over a hundred books and articles on the topic to learn everything I could about how hormones impacted weight loss, how to get tested, and what treatment options were available. I loaded myself up with information, found a hormone doctor, and successfully balanced my hormones for weight loss.

Learning about health and nutrition is how the miracle of weight loss begins. It is time to get excited about learning what will lead to greater weight-loss success. Start buying books and magazines that inspire you to eat clean, work out, or master the mental. Read success stories like the ones in this book and other inspiring stories of weight-loss success. This will inspire you to want the same thing in your own life. Follow in the footsteps of winners.

### 3. Remove energy vampires from your life.

Energy vampires are people whose mere presence or conversation drains or sucks the life out of you. Energy vampires suck away all the positive energy from your life. Some people are not kind, nice, or supportive and you should minimize or eliminate the time you spend with them. Some of us have family members and friends ruining our self-esteem every day. Even if they are your flesh and blood, try to remove yourself from their presence as much as possible. Hurtful words negate any progress toward self-worth and self-love. If you have a plan or vision for your life, you have to guard your mind and spirit against negative critics and energy vampires.

I am always monitoring my energy level around certain people. If I feel my energy dipping or my mood saddening in someone's presence, I will limit my exposure to that person. Negativity, just like positivity, is contagious. Be sure you are attracting positive energy in your life at all times. I love myself and the vision I have of my life too much to let negative, bitter, or small-minded people discourage me. I can transform any conversation with anyone to a place of positivity and enlightenment because my life and success depend upon it.

### 4. Create mini-habits to learn consistency.

Losing weight requires a new set of habits. Your past habits are the reason you are at your current undesirable weight. So, you will need different habits in order to get a different result. Because it is easy to revert back to old habits, creating new ones will be like creating a fortress that is strong and reliable and will help you minimize setbacks on your journey.

A mini-habit is a small action or behavior that you do every day that is designed to help you achieve lasting change by ensuring consistent action over time. It can be so small and simple that it can take less than a minute to complete. The body and brain change best at a slow pace over time so the mini-habits align to help you achieve lasting change.

Examples of daily mini-habits include:

- Read one chapter in a book.
- Listen to one song that inspires you.
- Drink one green smoothie.
- Do ten jumping jacks.

You may feel like you can do more, and of course you can, but by making it so ridiculously simple, you can get to a point where you always do it without fail. When you always do something, you become unstoppable, plain and simple.

The best way to know if you have created a good mini-habit is to think about whether you can still do it on your worst, most unproductive day. If you can succeed in doing your mini-habit on your worst day, then you will not fail. You'll also feel inspired by your consistency and naturally increase the habit day after day, week after week. If the habit was to do ten jumping jacks, you may find yourself doing fifty or a hundred in no time. However, you are only required to do the mini-habit each day. Having a low requirement, but exceeding it every day, is great for mastering consistency. It propels your upward potential toward greater habits, which leads to greatness in your life.

### 5. Create obstacles to avoid temptation.

You always have a choice in everything. You have options. I remember when I used to work in an office, I would go to unhealthy restaurants with friends at lunch every day. Each morning, I would say, I am eating healthy today or I am bringing a healthy lunch. But as soon as lunchtime came around, I went to eat at unhealthy restaurants with my friends. Eventually, I made the decision to eat healthy at least three days a week to accelerate my weight loss. So, I started to schedule my meetings closer to lunchtime so I would not have time to go out to lunch. This would keep me stuck and not able to go out to lunch with my friends at least three days a week. This worked better for me, and I was able to get more work done and get out of there on time each evening. This was helpful because no matter how many times I packed lunch for myself and carefully planned my meals, my friends at work would sabotage my efforts. That was not their intention, but even those who love and care for you do not always support you day in and day out. Be sure you have a plan to avoid obstacles and temptations that you encounter each day. Another way to achieve this is to do your grocery shopping online to avoid impulse buys when you walk the aisles.

### 6. Get someone in your household to hold you accountable.

Our eating habits are greatly influenced by our culture and by family and friends. Think about the people you eat with most often: loved ones, friends, and lovers. For a lot of us, food equals fun. We eat to socialize, celebrate, and show love to one another. How many people can say they eat right until they get around their family and friends? Our family and friends have the strongest influence on how successful we will be in changing our habits and living a healthy lifestyle. They often encourage us to indulge or tell us we look good and do not need to be on a diet. Whenever we tell someone we love that we are making some changes and getting healthier, their response will have a large effect on whether we succeed or fail.

Studies show that people who do not get support from loved ones are less successful in achieving their life goals. When you communicate to a family member that you are trying to lose weight, it is essential that they understand that your new lifestyle is important to you and show support and encouragement. If they do the opposite, or criticize your food choices, you will have a harder time succeeding, and this disagreement will become a source of stress and tension in the relationship. The ideal situation is when a family member decides to change their behavior along with you. That way, you can hold each other accountable. That way, if they challenge you and say "we" are not exercising enough, then you will not feel bossed around because they are speaking for the both of you. This kind of support will not feel condescending or judgmental and will increase your chance of success.

### 7. When you have to eat unhealthy foods to avoid hurting people's feelings, eat only small amounts.

For many families, food equals fun. Food is love, and food is how family shows love to one another, so when you change your eating habits and do not eat some of the things you used to, family can feel rejected because you turned down a meal or dessert. And if it's Momma who made it just for you and you turned it down, she can feel like you rejected her, not just the food. The solution is to use time with family as a cheat meal. That way, you can enjoy a festive family function without hurting anyone's feelings. Now you could say, it is too bad if their feelings are hurt, but I am going to do what is best for me, and that may work fine for you. However, for me, if Aunt Judy shows her love by baking a sweet potato pie, I'm gonna eat it and show her how much I appreciate her.

But what you can do to not go off track is to eat only a few spoonfuls of the unhealthy foods. There is no reason to go overboard, just take enough to enjoy the dish and show appreciation for a home-cooked meal made with love just for you. At the end of the day, the goal is to enjoy your family without totally sabotaging the progress you have made. Be sure to appreciate and love family and friends and make sure those emotions are directed at the person not just toward the food.

### 8. When you have to eat fast food, choose the healthy options on the menu.

There are times when you only have a few minutes to grab a meal and fast food restaurants may be your only option. So, do not be afraid of drive-thru or fast food restaurants—they are not an automatic no. Most fast food restaurants have healthy options. For breakfast, choose oatmeal; for lunch and dinner, there are usually healthy salads and wraps. It is all about choices. You just need to choose the healthy option. Salads with meat in them will give you the right balance of carbs and proteins. This is great news because a lot of us use our hectic schedule as an excuse to eat unhealthy. Just choose wisely, get a quick, healthy meal, and keep it moving.

### 9. When in a fancy restaurant, do whatever you can to make your food healthier.

This is a tricky one because oftentimes a date wants to take you to a nice restaurant, and the best restaurants typically have the most unhealthy meal options. You will have to be prepared to improvise. For example, you can ask for sauces and toppings on the side and use them sparingly. Additionally, the new trend is for restaurants to offer a low-calorie or "skinny" option on the menu. But as a general rule of thumb, high-end restaurants are all about the special preparation of sauces (often creamy) and seasonings (often salty) by a chef more concerned with flavor than healthfulness. If you are on a date with a romantic partner, offer to share appetizers or large entrees. Make the meal a shared romantic exploration without either of you eating too much.

### 10. Have snack options ready for those afternoon cravings.

Doesn't it seem that everyone gets hungry in the afternoon? That period between lunch and dinner can seem like forever. Not only that, but energy dips in the afternoon, particularly if you had a light lunch. You could also just be crashing because you are sleep-deprived. Before you wander to the vending machine, first have a glass of water, which will make you feel fuller. Then, depending upon how hungry you still are, have healthy

snacks handy. Healthy snack choices that will energize you include apples and peanut butter, nuts and seeds, hummus, or
protein bars. What if you forget to bring your own snacks?
Then try to choose the best options from the vending
machine—such as, lightly salted popcorn, peanuts, etc. Avoid
high-sugar snacks like cookies and candy bars.

### 11. When you consume alcohol, forego the mixers.

Oftentimes, even weekly for some, we find ourselves at a happy
hour with friends and coworkers. The important thing to remember is that the mixers—sodas, juices, and other mixers—
are what make cocktails so calorie-rich and unhealthy. A better
option is to have liquor on the rocks or neat, with no chasers.
Now, in general, alcohol is not the healthiest thing to put in
your body, but it doesn't mean it has to be avoided altogether.
Choose lower-calorie cocktails, such as gin, tequila, and tonic
or cognac and a diet coke and enjoy yourself.

## CONCLUSION

Now for your homework: Identify at least three success habits
that you can implement in your life right away. Do not just rely
on your willpower and self-control to lose weight. Think about
how you can control your environment to minimize temptations and distractions. Over time, these success habits will naturally lead to more long-term success.

# 11

## Have a Support System in Place

E VER WONDER WHY more than 60 percent of adults in the United States are overweight when there are so many diet plans, gadgets, and gyms available? There are many reasons, but one of the most important ones is that too few people understand the value of having a support system on their weight-loss journey. Having accountability partners keeps you on track and leads you down the road to successful, long-term weight loss.

There are some people who make up their mind to lose weight all on their own, but they are few and far between. If you are like me, you are not the type who can go it alone. Your support system can be a friend, family, spouse, coworker, or even a social media community. Whenever I fall off track, I go right to my Facebook community to get encouraged, motivated, and focused. I know almost everything about weight loss, but I still need extra support and encouragement when life gets hectic and stressful.

# WHAT ARE THE BENEFITS OF A SUPPORT SYSTEM?

## *Accountability*

It is easy to break promises to yourself to eat better and exercise. But when you are checking in with the people in your support group, you are more likely to stick to your weight-loss routine. A support system keeps you accountable to your weight-loss goals and will help you stay focused, strong, and sensible.

Since 95 percent of dieters fail within a year and more than 70 percent of gym-goers quit in less than three months, you are going to have to do some things differently if you want long-term success. Studies show that people enjoy exercise more when they do it with a friend because it feels more like socializing. The boredom of exercising is replaced by the fun of talking to a friend.

## *Gets You Through the Rough Times*

When your energy or motivation is low, sometimes you need an extra push. This is perfectly normal, so plan for these type of setbacks. Having a workout partner or any type of support system will keep you from falling off. A friend will catch you before you fall and encourage you to get back on the program quickly. Think of your time with a workout partner like an appointment. Even though people break promises to themselves all the time, rarely do they miss appointments. No one really wants to let someone down. You will feel much more compelled to keep your appointment when someone is counting on you.

## *Sets Up a Collective Goal*

You want people in your support system who understand your goals, people who will help motivate you when you feel like giving up. By having partners who support you, you will not be alone. You will have cheerleaders and mentors picking you up when you fall and helping you every step of the way. You all have a common, collective goal and remain committed to one another in achieving it.

The relationships you have during your weight-loss journey will be critical to getting to your goal weight. Even if you have tried before and failed, having someone there for support makes all the difference in the world. If you are dealing with a tough emotional situation or late-night boredom eating, talking to someone about your challenges improves your odds of succeeding.

Think about how it would be if you decided to build an extra room on your house. Think about how much time it would take, given all the mistakes you would make because you are not a builder/contractor. You have not learned the craft or the tricks to be successful in building a new room. You would have to get a coach or an expert to guide you through the process to ensure success. Without the expert, imagine how many times you would have to stop, restart, and make adjustments to get back on track.

Now imagine how much time, effort, and money you could save by simply having that expert with you right from the beginning. This person could be teaching you, cheering you on when you make progress, and helping you avoid pitfalls to keep you moving forward.

Similarly, it is difficult to lose weight on your own. This is why having the support of a coach is just as important on your weight-loss journey. A coach could be a fitness trainer, a weight-loss expert, or an online community that is a virtual weight-loss coaching program. Staying close to a group of folks who have gone down that road themselves or someone who has coached hundreds of people to lose weight before you will greatly increase your chance of getting to your ideal weight. They will provide lots of motivation, inspiration, and the proper tools, knowledge, and guidance along the way.

## WHY A WEIGHT-LOSS SUPPORT SYSTEM CAN MAKE THE DIFFERENCE FOR SUCCESS

Over the past couple of years, I have helped millions of people lose weight. I have seen great success for some, but for others, not much progress. Losing weight really can be a difficult goal to accomplish for some people.

A great benefit of having the support of family and friends is that they can benefit too. One study found that friends and family of overweight people who lose weight also lost weight themselves. By supporting a loved one or friend trying to lose weight, you will likely begin a better lifestyle for yourself!

## CREATING YOUR CIRCLE OF INFLUENCE

You will have your greatest success at weight loss when you surround yourself with like-minded people working toward the same goal. They will understand your journey, what you are doing, why you are doing it, and the challenges you are going through, and they can support and motivate you along the way.

It is important to create a circle of influence that is filled with positive, supportive people. They should have a winner's mind-set and a "can-do" attitude. They should be people who will lift you up and not tear you down. They should be people who will listen but accept no excuses from you.

It is not enough just to have a support system around you, you have to take action and utilize them. You have to share your goals with them and ask that they support you as you work toward those goals. If your spouse and children are a part of your support system, it is important to let them know exactly what your goals are so they do not inadvertently sabotage you. If your husband constantly brings home cookies and ice cream, and you are struggling to resist them, try making a plan to keep the treats out of the house or have your husband not eat them in front of you. You will need the support of the people closest to you to increase your chance of success.

It can also be fun to have the support of an online support community, new virtual friends with whom you can learn from as well as make mistakes and overcome challenges together. They can share with you what has worked for them and what has not and keep you highly motivated.

Here are some tips for leveraging a support system to help you lose weight:

- *Take a few minutes to think about what support you need on this journey.* Use a journal to write down a few notes and be as specific as possible so your family members know how best to support you. An example would be, "Eat junk foods in a different room than where I am." This will allow family members to have a better understanding of how to support you.

- *Communicate your goals with your family.* This will allow them to hold you more accountable. As an example, if your goal is to stop eating candy and sweets, then your family can help you avoid them when you're home or out in public.
- *Keep unhealthy foods out of sight.* Ask your family members to keep their unhealthy foods in a place (garage, cabinet, room) where you will not see them. If the foods are not visible, you will feel less tempted by them. Out of sight, out of mind.
- *Tell your family and friends to not give you food as a gift!* Explain to them that when a person trying to lose weight is given food as a gift, the temptation can be very difficult to overcome as cravings increase.

I hope these tips help you to create a supportive environment that allows for success. Everyone needs support and encouragement to achieve his or her goals in life, so be proactive about maintaining a supportive environment.

## SO HOW DO YOU CHOOSE A SUPPORT SYSTEM?

So many people put effort into finding the right exercise or weight-loss plan, but do not put any energy into creating their support system. But as we have seen, this support system is crucial, and it is worth putting some thought into setting up the best system to ensure your success.

Do not assume that your closest family member or friend is the best source of support. Think very deeply and be brutally honest about who has been helpful to keep you on track in the past.

The ultimate support system will be made up of people who have a common goal of getting slimmer and healthier and are committed to doing whatever it takes to achieve it. This could include working out together, cooking together, meal-prepping together, sharing recipes, grocery shopping or just touching base on the phone weekly. It really depends on what support you actually need. Encouragement can come in many forms. Some folks just need a motivational word or quote each day to stay on track.

Consider your support person's availability. Discuss how much time and energy you both have to devote to the partnership and how realistic it is to be available to support one another. At this time, discuss the primary mode of contact and support. Determine if you prefer phone, email, or text communications, this will be key to maintaining contact. Everyone likes to communicate in different ways. If you really need more face-to-face time, discuss that as well and figure out the best times to achieve it. The goal is to ensure that there is time devoted to listening and encouraging each other.

We touched on having a support community, and social media groups can be a good way to maintain success and get the support you need. Online support communities on social media help you to maintain accountability and get the encouragement you need. Whatever form of support you prefer, make sure to set up your support system very early on in your journey.

## THE BUDDY CONTRACT

Something that is becoming popular in the weight-loss community is the "buddy contract." This is a document that spells out the mutual goals of two people and the ways they plan to help each other achieve them, as well as a mode of communication.

The buddy contract should include both short-term goals (such as, "Meet at the gym three times a week to work out together") and long-term ones (such as, "My goal is to lose 120 pounds to achieve my ideal weight"). Just make sure the goals are specific and achievable.

Once you write up your buddy contract, you can both maintain a copy of the agreement and post it somewhere so you can reread it often and be reminded of what you are trying to accomplish.

Reevaluate your buddy relationship from time to time to ensure that it is working for both of you. Do not be afraid to call it quits if the relationship is not working out. Just like with any relationship, if you are not getting what you need, have a heart-to-heart with your buddy and either work to fix or end the buddy relationship. The purpose of the relationship is to enhance the weight-loss journey and make it easier to achieve your goals. If that is not happening, no need to force the relationship. In most cases, the support buddy relationship can blossom into a beautiful friendship for many years, so enjoy it. You may be building a lifelong friendship that continues for the rest of your life.

## CONCLUSION

Long-term weight loss is about changing behaviors and habits, which is very challenging. Having a support system in place will help you keep going when you feel like quitting. Your support system makes celebrating your successes more rewarding and fulfilling. It is also more fun celebrating with others. Your support system also encourages you to continue healthy eating and keeps you lifted up when you struggle. It will remind you that you are not alone and will make the journey more enjoyable and successful.

# 12

## Supercharge Your Spiritual Life

WE KNOW THAT there is more to weight loss than nutrition and exercise. Sticking to a diet regimen and ultimately making lifestyle changes to lose weight permanently are the outcomes of how we feel, what we think, and the actions we consistently take. The main problem is not your physical weight but what is happening in your mind and spirit, causing you to gain weight. Until your mind and spirit are engaged in your weight-loss efforts, excess weight will continue to be a problem for you. In this chapter, you will learn that who you are spiritually drives how you feel, what you think, and hence the actions you take in your life. I hope to give you a fresh perspective on spirituality without regard to religion so you can better apply positive spiritual practices to your life that not only support weight loss, but also accelerate and virtually guarantee it!

I coach thousands of people to weight-loss success every

year. To that end, I spend countless hours creating content and programs designed to help people lose weight, get healthier, and grow in confidence and self-esteem. This is my life's work. I am passionate about helping people get to the next level in their lives. I cannot begin to express the pure joy I feel when I see people transform their lives.

In fact, everyone on my team and especially my best friend knows this. When I see a particularly dramatic transformation photo or receive a success story by email, I immediately call him. If he does not answer right away, I keep calling. I am literally bubbling over with joy and have to share the good news. And of course, I always want him and everyone else that hears their success story to be as overjoyed as I am. This is the work that I feel called to do at this point in my life, so I experience pure joy when I see others achieving their weight-loss goals.

How do I know I am called to do this work? Well, I love what I do. I am really good at it. I get a great deal of internal joy from it. My life's journey has led me to this work and more important, it has been confirmed in my Spirit. Whoa! Confirmed in my Spirit? What does that mean? Well, it is a deeply personal, soul-based feeling that I feel connected to. I have a sense of responsibility for it and feel like it has what I am supposed to be doing on this earth.

I am a Christian woman with a deep faith in Christ. A more accurate description of who I am is "I love God, but I just cuss a little and listen to lots of hip-hop." I was raised in the church, sang in the choir, and taught Sunday school for years. However, I did not find my calling in the Scriptures. It was not written anywhere that I am supposed to help hundreds of thousands of people around the world lose weight and get healthy. That is what I discovered as part of my own unique spiritual journey.

## MY JOURNEY TO SPIRITUALITY

I grew up with the best Mom and Dad a child could ever ask for. Unfortunately, my dad passed away over twenty-five years ago. I wish I could introduce you to my dad. He taught me everything about competing, winning, learning, and being proud of who I am and where I came from. He was athletic, smart, confident, generous, humble, and deeply spiritual. He loved and served his community and you would be hard pressed to find anyone who did not both like and admire him.

When I went to college, it was one of the happiest times in my life. I had many natural gifts, had worked hard in high school, and graduated at the top of my class. I tested well on my SATs and had the option to go to just about any college that I wanted, including Ivy League schools. But through campus visits and consultation with my mom and dad, I decided to attend Hampton University in southern Virginia. Hampton is a historically black college and university (HBCU) and though it might seem counterintuitive to attend an HBCU when you have an Ivy option, my parents knew it was the right school for me.

In the midst of getting settled in and making new friends, my family discovered the unthinkable. My dad had been diagnosed with prostate cancer, which prompted my own initial deep study of health and wellness. I looked into anything that I thought would help my dad get well! I studied alternative medicine and any available treatments for his cancer. Of course, I wanted desperately to learn ways to help my dad. My attempts were futile and so were those of the numerous doctors and family members. My dad passed away the day I graduated from Hampton University.

After my dad died, I had to figure out how a man "so good" and "so needed" could be taken away from our family so soon. I had to deal with a devastating personal loss of my dad, who I loved with all my heart. I admired him and wanted to be like him and make him proud of me. There is still not a day that goes by that I do not feel deeply connected to him. I would love to hear him laugh again, see him hit a golf ball, or have him see who I have become today.

None of the Sunday school classes I had taught, sermons I had heard, or funeral services I had attended prepared me to handle the loss of my dad. I knew my dad lived "right" and was going to heaven, but no words or logic could console me. This would be something that I had to experience for myself, which sparked a deeper, more personal spiritual journey. Ultimately, I hung on to everything he taught me, but especially his last words to me. He said, "God is real. Seek Him and get to know Him for yourself." For me, this was the start of a deeper spiritual journey that caused me to transcend my thinking and grow spiritually beyond my religious practice and culture.

This chapter is not about religion. It is about spirituality and my establishing a strong spiritual foundation. Who I am spiritually does not compete or conflict with my religious beliefs. It only serves to reconcile who I am as an individual and how to actively apply my religious beliefs to my life.

Spirituality escapes no one. Whether you subscribe to a specific religion, are agnostic, atheist, or claim to be nonspiritual, no one escapes it. Spirituality is a universal human experience regardless of your religious practices or religious denials: the primary purpose of who you are as a spiritual being will be considered, contemplated, and resolved for you at some point in your life.

## SO, WHAT IS SPIRITUALITY?

Spirituality is not religion, but religion can be a spiritual experience for many. Spirituality does not have to be religious or tied to any particular theology, practice, or deity. Spirituality is inclined to be more personal and private whereas religion tends to be more corporate, and organized with specific doctrines and rituals.

Religion can be defined as the belief in and worship of a higher power, usually a God or gods based on faith, with some organizational structure governed by a set of doctrines, habits/rituals, and practices. Whereas spirituality refers to an inner path enabling a person to discover the essence of their being. Spirituality includes a sense of connection to something bigger than ourselves, and it typically involves a search for meaning in life. It is about becoming the best version of yourself in the areas of health, love, relationships, purpose, and community.

Initially, much of our spirituality is shaped by our religious ideology. As we reconcile our theology with what sits well in our spirit, we become more enlightened and develop spiritually. Even if you do not subscribe to a particular religion, you still must reconcile and embrace who you are as a spiritual being. There are universal questions that everyone must answer for themselves, often without regard to their religious beliefs.

What is my purpose? What is the meaning of life? How am I connected in the world? Is there such thing as a one true love? Questions like these are examples of those universal questions that must be discovered on your own unique spiritual journey. You may hear many religious or intellectual discussions that attempt to answer many of these questions, but they will not matter until you accept "the" answers in your spirit and store them deep within your soul.

Who we are spiritually rarely fails us, but what we feel can be easily negotiated or ever changing, like the wind. In an earlier chapter, we talked about how resistance prevents us from achieving our life purpose, dreams, and goals. What we believe intellectually is always open to debate as new information is made available to us all the time. How we reason, remember things, and solve problems are all controlled by the front part of our brain called the cerebrum. The cerebrum is designed to change. In fact, there is a relatively new area of study called neuroplasticity, which deals with the brain's ability to change at any age as we learn, forget, and age.

What we believe in our spirit lives in a deeper more sacred and protected place: our soul. What we believe deeply, we are more connected to. This goes beyond our intellect. It is the internalization of our beliefs and why we believe them. Our soul is the spiritual part of us that is distinct from the physical self. It cannot be observed or monitored. What we feel in our spirit can often defy logic.

When I decided to become an author, I had a great job. I was an executive and partner in an IT management consulting firm, made great money, and was admired by my team and customers. I was often referred to as the Michael Jordan of consulting because of my ability to execute. Why would anyone leave that for the uncertain life of an author? I had no platform, had never written any books, and had never thought of making a living as an author. However, it was something that I had to pursue. I knew it deep within my spirit.

Every day I would say, "I have to change my life." Many

would look at me, confused when they heard me say it, but I did not need their approval. I would just go back to laboring away on writing my book. They did not know, but I knew in my spirit that it was my time to do what would eventually lead me to my calling. No one else could know. It was a part of my own spiritual journey.

## SPIRITUALITY PAVES THE WAY TO WEIGHT-LOSS TRANSFORMATION

At the heart of every problem, including problems with your weight, is a spiritual problem. We lose our power to lose weight and keep it off because we are disconnected from our spirit and divine purpose in life.

If being spiritual is becoming the best version of ourselves and seeking our highest purpose in life, then it is supremely spiritual to want to be the healthiest version of ourselves and losing weight is an important part of that. Sure, there are many ways to achieve better health; build more muscle, improve our cardio, be better hydrated, and become more flexible, are just a few examples. These are all excellent things to do for better overall health and well-being, but the granddaddy of them all is to achieve and maintain a healthy body weight.

Being overweight is often a precursor to diseases that can kill or cripple you, including diabetes and metabolic syndrome, atherosclerosis, arterial plaque, cardiac arrest, pulmonary hypertension, and stroke. There are other conditions associated with carrying excess weight that simply hinder your overall health and ability to enjoy time with family and friends.

In addition to the physical issues associated with being overweight, there are a number of psychological and social issues too. Overweight and obese people are often targets of bias, stigma, and negative perceptions at work, school, and in interpersonal relationships.

As you embark upon your spiritual journey, it is important to realize that food cravings are a wake-up call to help us understand what we are truly craving in life. Most of our physical cravings lead us back to a craving for more meaning and purpose in life. Food becomes our comfort, our joy, and our peace, which leads to unhealthy eating and being overweight or obese. However, food can only fill your stomach, never your soul.

Spiritual maturity will help you realize that your true weight-loss goal is not a number on the scale. Your real weight-loss goal is peace. As much as I worshipped God, I turned to food in times of sadness, boredom, loneliness, stress, and even happiness. Now I just want peace over the struggle with my weight. Ironically, many churches feed our food addiction by using food for fellowship, not realizing that they are sabotaging many of us with unhealthy food choices.

For me, exercising consistently is a big challenge. However, the more I make exercising about spiritual growth, the less I focus on weight loss. Same with eating. Every time I wanted to eat when I was not physically hungry, I would ask myself if I was feeling spiritually hungry. With each pound I lost, I looked at it as a journey not to get slim but to grow spiritually. I began focusing on the spiritual goal of breaking free from the control of food rather than the physical goal of losing weight.

Scientists are now telling us what we already know. We've already been told by wise men, spiritual leaders, and our parents since the beginning of time that having a stronger connection with your God (in my case) and for others, Allah, Buddha, or the universe, will help you live longer and better.

Science has found that people who have strong spiritual practices are more resistant to health problems and actually live longer. Giancarlo Lucchetti, MD, PhD, is a researcher and scientist focused on spirituality and health. He is the lead author of a study that calculates that the life-lengthening benefits of spirituality can be compared to eating a high amount of fruits and vegetables or even taking blood pressure medication. This validates that a stronger spiritual foundation is key to a healthier life.

As you can imagine, doing a study to measure a person's spirituality is difficult. After all, how do you measure what is in a person's soul? However, most researchers agree that there is a positive relationship between good spiritual practices and better health outcomes.

A good spiritual practice specifically aids in weight loss by lowering stress, which reduces cortisol levels and reduces fat storage. It improves mental clarity and creates a higher commitment to tasks, which makes it easier for you to do what you planned and know how to do. Being healthy and strong spiritually will allow you to win in the battle against emotional eating because it improves the overall feeling of self-fulfillment and makes it easier to accept and deal with negative emotions.

It is great that science confirms our spiritual teachings, but the real confirmation should come from a place deep in your soul: your Spirit! You should know in your soul that you are a special creation with a unique purpose and connection to this world. It is your own personal spiritual journey to discover your life's meaning and purpose so that you can live your very best life.

## HOW TO ACHIEVE A STRONGER SPIRITUAL FOUNDATION FOR WEIGHT LOSS

There are a number of ways to tap into a greater level of spirituality. These practices apply to both those that are religious and those that are not. Religion does not conflict with these spiritual practices. For example, regardless of your religion, everyone can benefit from becoming more enlightened through study and quieting of the mind. Visualization, connecting with nature, art, and music are good for everyone's soul.

Described below are various categories of ways to reach a higher level of spirituality. Some of them you will already be engaged in on a regular basis and others you will want to consider adding, as they will help you better connect to yourself and the world. This is by no means an exhaustive list, but will get you started and will have a positive impact on your weight-loss journey and overall well-being.

- *Contemplative* activities can promote deep, reflective thinking. Examples are meditation, prayer, journaling, visualization, and spending time alone. These are practices that connect you to your inner soul and bring you a sense of peace and promote clarity. As an example, you can start the day with prayer, meditation, or self-reflection.
- *Enlightenment* involves learning new ideas for the advancement of the individual. Examples would include reading Scriptures, deep study, and reading inspirational books.
- *Physical* involves any physical activity that requires movement by the body or physical exertion by your

muscles. Examples include yoga, martial arts, exercise, or walking.

- *Nature* does wonders for the soul. When we spend time in nature, we are reminded that life is fleeting and sometimes we need that perspective in order to remember what truly matters. Additionally, views of the water, sunrises and sunsets, and mountain ranges all have a calming effect for most.

- *Music/Arts* inspire spiritual expression. Music and the arts are a creative expression that have a profound impact on the mind by allowing a person to connect with a deeper part of themselves.

- *Fellowship* is more than merely a time to get together for various activities and food. Every fellowship event offers an opportunity to connect with like-minded folks who are also trying to grow spiritually. It allows you to connect with others, interact, experience, observe, become more tolerant, learn, and share with others who are also on a journey to grow spiritually.

- *Acts of kindness* pave the way for spiritual growth. It allows you to show the tender mercy and kindness of God. Examples include volunteering, giving, or charity work of any kind.

## CONCLUSION

The standard ways of addressing weight loss have too often failed or had fleeting results, so it is time to look for a deeper approach for long-term success. We have learned that good spiritual practices have such a positive impact on our health and weight, so by addressing spirituality as a necessary tool for weight loss, you are dealing with the root cause of why you have struggled with your weight for so long. You have to assess and apply good spiritual practices that work to support weight loss, healthy living, and happiness.

Permanent weight loss is a transformative experience because it is a spiritual battle, not just a physical one. For many of us, we truly need a miracle to get this weight off because we have tried every diet and weight-loss plan out there. You can break free of your unhealthy eating habits. Today, I feel I have a good relationship with food. I can have ice cream in my refrigerator and not eat it for weeks. I do not overindulge nor do I deny myself the ice cream, because the food is never the real issue. I give myself permission to eat unhealthy food from time to time and to enjoy it.

You can lose excess weight once and for all. By doing the spiritual work, along with changing your habits and your environment, eating clean food, and incorporating good exercise habits, you have no reason not to achieve your ideal weight. This is your new beginning. You are no longer the same person you used to be. Your mind and body are no longer the same. Always honor the spirit, and the mind and body will follow.

# Part Three

---

## 30-DAY
## MENTAL
## MASTERY
## CHALLENGE

Part 3, 30-Day Mental Mastery Challenge, provides thirty days of exercises supporting the strategies taught in the SUCCESS System to ensure you can create new habits and behaviors that create lasting and permanent weight loss for life. These thirty exercises will help you get your mind right, strengthen your mental focus, and overcome bingeing and emotional eating so that you can get to your goal weight once and for all.

# 13

# 30-Day Mental Mastery Challenge

O NE OF THE most important things folks need for long-term weight-loss success is Mental Mastery. Dieters know that there is more to weight loss than "eat less and exercise," and this book provides the missing piece they need to win at weight loss once and for all. In this book, we teach dieters the SUCCESS System, seven mental strategies required for permanent weight loss.

The 30-Day Mental Mastery Challenge provides thirty days of exercises supporting the strategies taught in the SUCCESS System. This will ensure that you create new habits and behaviors that create lasting and permanent change allowing you to maintain a healthy weight for life. These thirty exercises will help you process toxic emotions, strengthen your mental focus, and overcome emotional eating so that you achieve your desired weight.

Although the path to losing weight is much more than a 30-

day plan, I want you to apply the strategies and solutions in the SUCCESS System so you have a foundation to create and maintain a whole new way of living and relating to food and your body.

The purpose of this challenge is simple: to be a wake-up call that will challenge those who are committed to getting slim and healthy. The exercises and strategies in this 30-Day Challenge will help you produce specific, measurable, long-lasting changes in yourself so that you can live the life of your dreams.

**WHAT YOU NEED TO COMPLETE THE 30-DAY MENTAL MASTERY CHALLENGE:**
1. *Journal* (to capture your thoughts and feelings)
2. *Pen/pencil* (to write down your thoughts and feelings)
3. *Open heart* (to be honest about mistakes you have made in the past)

## DAY 1: LOVE ME SOME ME (THE MIRROR EXERCISE)

*Food for thought:* Loving yourself first sends a clear message that you are to be recognized, celebrated, appreciated, and loved.

### *Exercise:*

Self-love is key to maintaining your healthy, ideal weight. The body has a natural ability to create and maintain the perfect weight for you as long as you are aligned with your true self.

Begin by standing in front of a mirror and looking deeply into your own eyes. Ask yourself if there is something you see there that you like. Can you look deeply into your own eyes and see yourself as God sees you? Can you see beyond your physical appearance? Can you accept the person you see in the mirror?

As you stare at yourself in the mirror, say the following affirmations:

1. I will do my best to love and respect my body. My body is a gift and deserves to be treated with love and kindness. I am sorry for the pain that I have caused you.
2. I am beautiful inside and out. I am perfect in this moment as I continue to move toward accepting myself.
3. My body deserves love. My body deserves to be respected. My body has gone through a lot and continues to carry me through, and for that I am grateful.
4. I will choose to help my body stay healthy by nurturing it with self-love, healthy food, and consistent exercise.
5. I know that this journey is a struggle, but I am going to try hard and do the best I can.

The point is to focus on self-love and self-acceptance and let go of what you believe other people think of you. In doing this, you have so much more power. You cannot control how other people perceive you. In fact, it has nothing to do with you—it is in their hands. However, you can control how you perceive yourself and you can control how you care and love for yourself. In doing this, you embrace your own power.

## DAY 2: KNOW YOUR WEIGHTS

*Food for thought:* Know that there is more than one number on the scale that can make you feel accomplished.

### *Exercise:*

Be careful of how you view the scale as it's just a data point, a tool to determine your physical weight, but it has no measurement for determining your worth. Do you get on your scale, hoping for a certain number to appear? If that number is not there, do you lose all motivation? If so, you may be setting yourself up for continual disappointment. Rather than focus on just one number, consider other ways to think about the numbers on the scale. In your journal, note the following:

1. *Dream weight:* A weight you would choose if you could weigh whatever you wanted.
2. *Happy weight:* This weight is not the one you'd choose as your ideal, but you'd be happy if you weighed only this much. You would still feel accomplished if you hit this weight.
3. *Acceptable weight:* A weight that would not make you particularly happy, but that you could be satisfied with or feel some sense of progress.
4. *Never-again weight.* The all-time high that you never want to hit again.

In your journal, jot down your dream weight, happy weight, acceptable weight, and never-again weight. Please note that you can also use dress sizes instead of weights. Then write down your actual weight/dress size, as of today. How many pounds is your real weight from your acceptable weight? Assuming you can lose two pounds a week, how many weeks would it take you to get to that weight?

In your journal, how do you envision yourself feeling and behaving once you reach your acceptable or happy weight? How about your dream weight? Do you have any plans once you reach your acceptable or happy weight, such as a shopping spree or a weekend trip? How will your life be different once you achieve your weight-loss goals?

## DAY 3: CREATE YOUR CIRCLE OF INFLUENCE

*Food for thought:* Surround yourself with like-minded, positive, supportive people who will help you achieve your weight-loss goals.

### Exercise:

You will have your greatest success at weight loss when you surround yourself with other like-minded people who are all working toward the same goal as you. Your chance of achieving your weight-loss goals greatly increases when you have people around you who understand your journey—what you are doing, why you are doing it, the challenges you are going through—and they can support and motivate you along the way. It is important to create a circle of influence that is filled with positive, supportive people. This circle of influence is called a support system and it is critical to your long-term success.

What kind of people should be in your circle of influence? Well, they should be motivational and supportive, with a winner's mind-set and "can-do" attitude. They should be people who will lift you up and not tear you down. They should be people who will listen but accept no excuses from you.

You will need the support of the people closest to you to increase your chance of success. It can also be fun to have the support of an online support community, new virtual friends who you can watch and learn from as well as make mistakes and overcome challenges with. They can share with you what has worked for them and what hasn't and keep you highly motivated.

Write down the names of the individuals (or online support groups) who are in your circle of influence. Make plans to share your goals with them and ask them for their support.


## DAY 4: CREATE POSITIVE AFFIRMATIONS

*Food for thought:* Allow your mind to work with your body to transform yourself, from the inside out.

### *Exercise:*

It's time to start communicating to your mind. Positive affirmations are positive phrases you repeat to yourself that describe how you want to be. You can use positive affirmations to create the change you desire in your life, whether that is weight loss, quitting smoking, or any bad habit. Since we are focusing on weight loss, below are some positive affirmations that focus on the change you want to create in your life. You should repeat these affirmations for two minutes daily so that every cell in your body can imagine them.

To begin loving your body and your true self, post the following affirmative statements on a note card or in your journal and read them every day before you leave for work or go to bed:

1. I will have a loving relationship with food. I know that food is a gift from God that I am grateful for because it nourishes my body.
2. I will not be afraid to get on the scale because the number I weigh isn't as important as the overall healthiness of my body. A healthy body is a beautiful body.
3. I will not be ashamed of my body, for it is just the house for my spiritual and mental self; it does not define my true self.
4. I will forgive myself and other people. No more arguing and fighting, only letting go of stresses, failures, and disappointments.
5. I am thankful for my body and look forward to a slimmer, healthier body as I become more enlightened about healthy eating.

## DAY 5: CREATE MINI-HABITS

*Food for thought:* When you do something consistently, you become unstoppable, plain and simple.

### *Exercise:*

Your current habits are the reasons behind your current weight. You will need different habits in order to get a different result. A mini-habit is a small action or behavior that you do every day. It can be so small and simple that it can take less than a minute to complete. The body and brain change best at a slow pace over time. A mini-habit is designed to help you achieve lasting change by ensuring consistent action over time. Because it's easy to revert to old habits, your mini-habits will be like a fortress that is strong and reliable, which minimizes setbacks on your journey.

Examples of mini-habits include:

1. Read one chapter in a book.
2. Listen to one song that inspires you each day.
3. Drink a green smoothie daily.
4. Do 10 jumping jacks every morning.

You may feel like you can do more, and of course you can, but by making it so ridiculously simple, you can get to a point where you always do it without fail.

The best way to know if you've created a good mini-habit is to think about whether you can still do it on your worst, most unproductive day. If you can, then you won't fail and you'll feel inspired by your consistency. You may start to naturally increase the habit day after day, week after week. If the mini-habit was to walk up one flight of stairs, you may find yourself walking up two or three in no time. However, you're only *required* to do the mini-habit each day. Having a low threshold, but exceeding it every day, is great for mastering consistency. It propels you toward even better habits, which lead to greatness in your life.

List five mini-habits you can focus on and begin just *one* today. Do it consistently for an indefinite period of time. You are learning to create lasting change in your life by mastering consistent action over time.

## DAY 6: LEARN TO COMMIT TO LOSING WEIGHT

*Food for thought:* Making sacrifices and putting in the necessary work takes commitment.

### Exercise:

Are you *interested* in losing weight or are you *committed* to losing weight? If you're truly committed, you'll do what it takes and make the necessary sacrifices to lose weight. People fail not because of lack of interest or desire but because of lack of commitment.

In your journal, write down at least five ways to show you are truly committed to losing weight, not just interested in doing so.

Examples: Have you let your friends and family know

you're committed to this journey? Have you changed your circle of friends to weed out naysayers and doubters? Have you bought a water pitcher for your desk so you can drink water more frequently? Are you reading about health and nutrition every day? Do you connect to your support system? Do you plan your meals each week to ensure you eat healthy?

## **DAY 7:** DEVELOP A FOOD-MOOD DIARY

*Food for thought:* It's not what you're eating, it's what's eating at you.

### *Exercise:*

For many of us emotional overeaters, it will take some time to really connect our experiences and our feelings with what we put into our mouths. It is a good idea to begin writing your food-feelings connections to give you more insights and awareness. When you write down every single thing that you eat, there is less chance of unconsciously eating something. This exercise will help you explore the connection between food and feelings.

Many of us are eating when we are not physically hungry. Do you eat when you are sad, bored, anxious, ashamed, angry, or afraid? Whenever you have an unpleasant feeling, do you use food to push away the feeling and sedate yourself? Some folks like crunchy foods when they are angry and sweets when they are bored and lonely. It's time to get in touch with how your feelings affect what you put in your mouth.

In your journal, create and complete the following Food-Mood Diary:

| Time | Food | Feeling Before | Feeling Afterwards |
|------|------|----------------|--------------------|
|      |      |                |                    |
|      |      |                |                    |
|      |      |                |                    |
|      |      |                |                    |
|      |      |                |                    |
|      |      |                |                    |

## DAY 8: HEAL A BROKEN HEART

*Food for thought:* Profound emotional sadness doesn't just weigh heavily on your mind, it can also significantly impact your body.

### *Exercise:*

Heartbreak can have a devastating effect on your health and particularly your weight. You can end up binge-eating or engaging in emotional eating to deal with the hurt and pain from a broken heart.

You have to choose to deal with the pain and not run from it or distract yourself from the pain by overeating. It's time to rise up to the challenge and deal with it head on. Some of us just keep jumping into new relationships to deal with a broken heart, but you will still have to process those emotions so they don't overwhelm you and linger with you for years.

Reflecting on past relationships (even if you're married) and looking at them as lessons learned can greatly enhance your ability to heal and move on. Some of us are in committed relationships now and still haven't processed painful feelings from past relationships.

In your journal, create and complete the following chart:

| Romantic Partner | How I Feel (One Word) | What I Learned From This Relationship |
| --- | --- | --- |
|  |  |  |
|  |  |  |
|  |  |  |
|  |  |  |
|  |  |  |
|  |  |  |
|  |  |  |
|  |  |  |
|  |  |  |
|  |  |  |

## DAY 9: ESTABLISH QUIET TIME WITH GOD

*Food for thought:* As we physically overeat, we are spiritually starving ourselves. We need to feed our spirit and starve the flesh from inappropriate eating.

*Exercise:*

---

It is important to establish quiet time, or spirit time, with your Lord, your divine, so that you can align your worldly self with your spiritual self. Creating a place in your home will help you establish a daily routine of prayer or self-reflection. This is a place where you cannot think so much about food but instead about your heart's desires, dreams, and goals. As you shift your thoughts toward having a stronger mind and spirit, your relationship with food will begin to shift and diminish.

Think about what area in your home would make a great place for prayer and self-reflection. Be sure there is room for a chair so you can sit and read the Word of God or other inspirational books, pray, and meditate. Decorate this area with your favorite objects, such as flowers, prayer beads, and pictures. This area should allow you to celebrate your desire to receive a miracle. This should be your dedicated space throughout your spiritual journey that allows you to focus on achieving your goals.

## DAY 10: SAY GOODBYE TO SADNESS AND HELLO TO JOY

*Food for thought:* Experiencing joy and happiness is your birthright.

*Exercise:*

---

**GOODBYE TO SADNESS:** By realizing that you have to make some changes to avoid emotional eating, you will have to acknowledge your losses. You will no longer be able to use food as a coping mechanism. Food is not to be used to make you feel better. Even though you may be more emotional than the next person, allowing your emotions to run your life has to end. No longer can you live in the vicious cycle of emotional overload, overeating, and self-loathing. Yes, you may feel sad and hurt sometimes, but overeating and bingeing not only leads to greater pain but also excess weight and poor health.

**SAY HELLO TO JOY:** When we're overwhelmed with sadness, hurt, and disappointment, joy seems so distant and far. We start to think that joy is something we won't ever feel again. But that is so far from the truth. Try to laugh, smile, and have a good time as often as you can. Life shouldn't feel burdensome, as though you're always caring for others and not caring for yourself enough. Commit to feeling pure joy more often. You have to learn what makes you happy and do whatever it takes to create those things in your life. Yes, you should do what makes you feel good. Experiencing joy and happiness is your birthright. Go for it. Go pursue happiness.

Now you will create two lists:

- Things that make me feel energized and happy
- Things that make me feel spontaneous and adventurous

Be sure to schedule at least one of these activities within the next few days.

**EXAMPLES OF THINGS THAT CAN MAKE YOU FEEL ENERGIZED AND HAPPY:**

1. Watch a funny movie that you know will make you laugh out loud.
2. Go out for drinks with old friends and laugh at life.
3. Play a game that makes you feel silly, like a kid.
4. Spend some time around children who encourage you to lighten up and be silly.

**EXAMPLES OF THINGS THAT CAN MAKE YOU FEEL SPONTANEOUS AND ADVENTUROUS:**

- Remodel and/or paint a room where you spend the most time with a color that soothes you.
- Take a hip-hop or salsa dancing class; maybe call a friend and ask them to join you.
- Pull your car over when you see a county fair and go enjoy it.
- Tag along with a friend to participate in an activity they enjoy. You may find that you like it too. If not, congratulate yourself for stepping out of your comfort zone and keep looking for other activities that make you happy.

**DAY 11:** SAY THIS PRAYER BEFORE EATING

*Food for thought:* Use the power of prayer by asking God to feed your hunger and heal your mind.

*Exercise:*

Every time you eat anything, say this prayer:

> *"God, feed my hunger and heal my mind. I need wisdom to make wise eating choices. I need power to walk away from temptations. Help me be free from the struggle with eating and weight gain. Allow me to find strength in Your love. In You, all things are possible. In Your Holy Name, Amen."*

Even if you are eating unhealthy food, say the prayer. God is not there to judge you but to restore you. This prayer will begin to dissolve the desire for unhealthy foods. And feel free to rewrite the prayer if there is something else you want to say.

## DAY 12: CREATE A "DO SOMETHING DIFFERENT" LIST

*Food for thought:* We have to deliberately identify new ways to deal with emotional, painful, or challenging situations that don't involve food or eating.

*Exercise:*

When you are overeating or binge-eating, you already know that it is bad for you and will work against your weight-loss goals. What will help you is learning new ways to cope with emotional, painful, or challenging situations that don't involve food or eating. We will explore different ways to cope that allow you to be more loving and kind to yourself.

As a coping mechanism to replace emotional eating, write

out a list of things that you can do to nurture yourself instead of indulging in unhealthy eating. This is called a "Do Something Different" List.

List as many alternatives to emotional eating as you can think of. Write the list on an inspirational notepad and keep it posted where you will read it when you need it the most.

Here are some examples of things that you can add to your "Do Something Different" List:

- Visualize something positive, like your next Caribbean vacation
- Lie down and rest or go to sleep, if tired
- Get out of your home or workplace and take a walk
- Download your favorite music and dance
- Call a friend, a family member, or a support buddy
- Go through magazines and clip art with which you'll create a vision board
- Go browse a bookstore or read a book
- Write a letter or journal entry in your diary
- Take out some art supplies and paint or draw or do scrapbooking
- Go to church/synagogue
- Watch a good movie or go out to the movies
- Relax in a detox bath
- Breathe/meditate/stretch/do yoga to focus on inner peace
- Bring food to homeless people in your neighborhood or to a local shelter

## **DAY 13:** DO A KITCHEN INVENTORY

*Food for thought:* Allow your kitchen to be a place for enjoying foods that fuel you.

### *Exercise:*

Go through the foods that you are likely to binge on or foods that you have binged on in the past. Ask a supportive person to come over and go through your cabinets and refrigerator with you. Get rid of all of those foods. If you live with a partner or spouse, you might need to sit down with them and explain to them what you're going through. This is really important. If you were an alcoholic, it would be crucial that your partner didn't bring alcohol into the house while you were going through recovery. Think of trigger foods like alcohol. You will feel more comfortable if they are not easily accessible. As you go on in your process, you might begin to learn new trigger foods that you never would have thought would cause you to binge.

For example, one client discovered that she couldn't keep raw, unsalted sunflower seeds in her home. If she did, she'd eat as many as she could and even if she finished them all, she would find something else to continue eating. Even though this was a healthy snack, it was a trigger food for binge eating.

Once you've cleared the house of binge foods, vow not to bring any binge foods home and declare your house a binge-free zone. This is not a forever thing, but for now, in the early parts of gaining control over your eating habits, you want to keep yourself safe. Just as a recovering alcoholic wouldn't spend time in a bar or keep bottles of gin in his or her home, you don't want to have any trigger foods in your home either.

You should also note in your journal all your trigger foods so you can stay away from them.

## DAY 14: FORGIVE YOURSELF AND OTHERS

*Food for thought:* If you want to release excess emotional weight, you will have to master forgiveness.

### Exercise:

There may be relationships in your present or past that have to be dealt with head-on in order to heal. Simply put, we have to forgive in order to lose excess weight.

First, list those whom you need to forgive but have not been able to forgive. Don't think we are just talking about grand things that you have to forgive; it can even be the slightest comment or annoyance from a coworker. It is anything that you have floating around in your mind that takes your thoughts away from God's love. It is not just the people who have deeply hurt or betrayed you. It can be people who have betrayed you in small ways as well. Whenever you think of their names, write them down in your journal as well as the feelings you have toward them. Take your time through the process so you can really feel your emotions toward each person. Say to yourself, "I am willing to forgive this person and see them the way God sees them." Sometimes you are forgiving a small thing, and sometimes it's a huge thing. But always know that forgiveness isn't your gift to them, it's your gift to yourself. Your emotional and physical weight will be released and you will feel lighter and freer to hear from God.

Don't overlook the opportunity to add yourself to the list of those you need to forgive. Most of us have done things we regret and feel guilty about. We may know that we have done somebody wrong and we have been carrying those feelings of guilt for years. Forgiving yourself is a critical part of the healing process.

Also, say to God, "I am sorry." Express what you are sorry for and who you are sorry to. If you have hurt someone else, they carry that in their spirit, but so do you as we are all connected to God's spirit. It may be necessary to reach out to that person to apologize even if it feels shameful or embarrassing. But your willingness to make amends for your past mistakes carries more power over losing weight than any diet plan on the market. Don't ignore your wrongdoings any longer. By hurting someone else, you have hurt yourself. Forgive today and forgive quickly so you can release emotional weight from your physical body.

## DAY 15: PLAN TO LOSE

*Food for thought:* All success in life starts with a plan.

### Exercise:

Ask winners the secret of their success in academics, business, or sports, and they consistently say they start with a plan. If you want to win the weight-loss war, you have to plan to lose weight. We suggest not just one master plan, but several plans. In your journal:

- *Make a weekly meal plan.* Every Sunday make a meal plan for the coming week. List the foods you need to buy on a grocery shopping list. My grocery shopping list is 80 percent the same each week.
- *Post this meal plan on your refrigerator door.* Check off each meal and day. If your eating doesn't go exactly according to plan, make adjustments as you plan the next day.
- *Plan for tomorrow.* Before you go to bed, make a healthy to-do list for the next day. Each night before bed, write down what you plan to eat the next day. Compliance experts know that if people actually put down on paper a list of what they intend to do, they're more likely to follow through. If you forgot to plan the night before, make up a menu in the morning, and stick to it so you aren't focusing on food later in the day when you're tired and hungry.
- *Now plan your indulgences.* List the foods you adore even though you know they aren't great for your weight loss or health. Rank your five favorites in order of their importance to you. Allow yourself to eat the top two or three but not the others. Plan how often (maybe start with just once per week) you will indulge. This allows you to enjoy meals/snacks that reward you for staying committed to your journey.

## DAY 16: WRITE A LETTER TO YOURSELF

*Food for thought:* You will need to do things differently in order to get a different result for your future.

### *Exercise:*

To improve all sorts of decisions in your life, you can get perspective from your past self to help you be more objective about your future. Writing a letter to your younger self can help you gain clarity and closure, forgive yourself and others, as well as heal hurts and pains.

Thinking about your past can be uncomfortable, but it's a healthy discomfort because you're confronting your own weaknesses and shortcomings. The goal is to help you reflect so you can make better decisions for your life in the future.

If you could go back fifteen years into the past, what would you tell your younger self? What lessons have you learned over the last fifteen years and how will those lessons help you be a smarter and wiser person going forward? Think about what things you would do differently if you had known better. What life lessons have you learned from your romantic relationships? What career opportunities did you miss because you were not qualified or you mismanaged your time at work? The reason we do this is because there's no use going another fifteen years repeating the same mistakes and setbacks in life.

In your journal, write the following:

*Dear Self,*

*I am coming to you from fifteen years in the future to give you some valuable information. Here's what I learned . . .*

## DAY 17: MEDITATE TO BUILD YOUR LIFE FOR TOMORROW

*Food for thought:* What we are today comes from our thoughts of yesterday, and our present thoughts build our life of tomorrow. Our life is the creation of our mind.

### Exercise:

Meditation quiets the mind, relaxes the body, and helps us to focus on the present. Once the head chatter has stopped, you are open to experiencing guidance or inner wisdom and might intuitively get an answer to a question that has plagued you.

Are you meditating at least once a day? Today's exercise focuses on meditating once today.

**HOW TO MEDITATE:** Although there are different types of meditation, most include the following:

- *Quiet.* Find a location without distractions (phone, TV, others talking) so you will not be disturbed.
- *Comfort.* You do not need to be sitting like a yogi to experience meditation. It is often recommended, however, that you keep your spine straight. If you tend to nod off, be seated rather than lying down.

- *Concentration.* You can gaze at an object (maybe one in nature—a leaf, waves of the ocean, a tree in the distance—or perhaps something like the flame of a candle).
- *Observation.* Rather than judging yourself, be in the role of a detached observer. No judgments, no criticisms, just notice with impartiality. Awareness of the breath.
- *Many meditations begin by placing your attention on your breathing.* As you do so, you become more and more relaxed. Inhale (count) through your nose. Pause. Exhale (count + 2) through your mouth. Pause. Repeat. Repeat. Repeat. Ignore thoughts and distractions, and continue to bring your awareness back to the breath.
- *Clear your mind.* Heighten your senses. Be still. Breathe. Meditate for 5 to 10 minutes.

## DAY 18: HAVE A MINDFUL MEAL

*Food for thought:* Learning the difference between physical hunger versus emotional hunger will help you gain control over your eating habits.

### Exercise:

The mindful meal is a planned meal in an intentional space that you create to understand more about your feelings when you are eating. It will help you focus on your own hunger, digestion, and moods. The more often you eat mindful meals, the better you will begin to understand the difference between real physical hunger and fake emotional hunger. Here are the steps:

**PREPARATION:**
- Set aside a time when you can be alone without any distractions.
- Turn off your television, computer, and phone.
- If you don't like dead silence, listen to light music.
- Make sure the lights are on and the room is well lit.
- Slowly and deliberately prepare a meal for yourself. Take time to notice the colors and smells of your food. Feel the sensation of cutting your vegetables and meat. Hear the sizzle of the food cooking but hold off on tasting anything until it's time to eat.
- Be sure not to eat any food or snack during the preparation phase. Do not eat until you are sitting at the table.
- Create a nice table setting for yourself. Use your favorite tablecloth, silverware, and dishes, and perhaps light some candles. You might also set out some flowers and make it beautiful for yourself.

**THE MEAL:**
1. Sit down. Before you begin to eat, assess how hungry you are.
2. Before you start to eat, look down at your food and see what is on your plate.
3. Take a breath and then say a word of gratitude, prayer, or grace.

4. Decide what you want to eat first and put that first forkful of food into your mouth. Chew it slowly and really taste it.

5. Continue to chew and taste the food thoroughly. Put your fork down after every two bites and pause.

6. Notice your thoughts and feelings as you eat. Notice how you feel when you are really focused on eating.

7. After you are halfway done with your meal, stop and put your fork down. Take a few deep breaths, close your eyes, and notice where you are on the hunger scale.

8. If you are still physically hungry and desire more food, allow yourself to eat more.

9. When you feel full and satisfied, put your fork down and place a napkin over your food.

10. Give yourself permission to get up from table, put your food away, and go do something else.

11. Notice what you are feeling. Are you satisfied? Do you want to eat more? Are you able to go do something else or are you thinking about eating more?

12. If you continue to think about food, even though you are not physically hungry, try to figure out what else is eating at you. What is it that you truly need right now?

13. If you continue to desire food, sit still, think for a while, and write in your journal what you are feeling. Allow your obsession with the food to pass so you can you enjoy some other activity besides eating.

Commit to having a mindful meal at least once a week to really help you tune in with your physical hunger and emotional hunger. It will help you be more conscious of your eating habits and your feelings and moods when you eat. As you continue on your journey, you will begin to gain more control over how to satisfy your body with food without overeating.

## DAY 19: CREATE A WEIGHT-LOSS VISION BOARD

*Food for thought:* Your mind responds strongly to visual stimulation.

### Exercise:

A weight-loss vision board is one of the most valuable weight-loss tools that can help you achieve your goals. If you want a vision of your future life to look completely different, then it's important to focus on the pictures and images that inspire you to make healthy choices along your journey.

Your mind responds strongly to visual stimulation, and when you surround yourself with images that invoke positive emotions, your brain will work to achieve the affirmations and images. Your vision board will program your subconscious to attract things that will help you reach your weight-loss goal.

**HOW TO USE YOUR WEIGHT-LOSS VISION BOARD:**
- Look at your vision board often to feel the inspiration it provides.
- Believe it is already yours.
- Read your affirmations and inspirational quotes out loud.
- See yourself living a life in your new slimmer body.
- Picture yourself shopping for smaller clothes.

**SUPPLIES TO MAKE YOUR VISION BOARD (YOU CAN ALSO CREATE AN ONLINE/VIRTUAL BOARD):**

- Pictures, quotes, and photos that cause happy thoughts (you can use magazines/books)
- Glue/pins, markers, scissors
- Poster board, a large sheet of paper, cork board, or pin board
- You can use glitter, paint, or stickers. It's your board. Make it your own.
- Have fun with it and get your children to help you.

**WHAT TO PUT ON YOUR VISION BOARD:**

- Pictures of how you want your body to look when you've lost weight
- Images, quotes, and words that give you happy thoughts
- Things you WANT to look at because they make you feel empowered, happy, and motivated about losing weight
- Motivational quotes that make you feel empowered
- Images of people you admire or people you love
- Pretty pictures of delicious food and healthy recipes you'd like to try
- The outfits you'll be wearing at your goal weight (skinny jeans and form-fitting dresses)
- A list of exercise goals—like crossing the finish line of a marathon or a Bikram yoga pose you'd like to master

When you complete your weight-loss vision board, be sure to share it with your friends, family, and online support system.

## DAY 20: LETTING GO OF CONTROL

*Food for thought:* In the process of letting go, you will lose many things from the past, but you will find yourself. —Deepak Chopra

### *Exercise:*

**LETTING GO OF CONTROL OF ANOTHER PERSON OR SITUATION.**

In your journal:

- Name a person or situation that is currently occurring that is causing you to feel powerless, hopeless, or out of control

- Is there any part of this situation that you can control? How can you do that? Which part do you have no control over?

- Admitting and understanding that you have no control over this person or situation, what can you do to soothe and take care of yourself?

- Write a letter to this person or to the situation letting them/ it know exactly what you're feeling. Don't hold back with this letter; let everything that you feel come out. Then, allow yourself to take the letter and burn it, or even put it in a bottle and send it out to sea, or pray and turn it over to God.

- Visualization Time: Imagine yourself on an island with the person or situation that feels out of control. See yourself saying goodbye to them or to the situation; then see yourself getting into a rowboat and rowing away. You see them and you wave goodbye as you continue to row your boat away from them. They continue to get smaller and smaller as you row farther and farther away. You know that the person or situation still exists, yet you are allowing yourself to detach from them. Realize that it might be beyond your power to solve or change this situation, so make a pact that you are going to stop trying. Instead, do something for yourself that feels good—detract attention from the person or situation and put that attention on yourself. Focus on what you do have control over and the power that you do have.

## DAY 21: SPEAK YOUR TRUTH

*Food for thought:* The first step in managing your emotional overload is to speak your truth unapologetically, without shame, fear, or embarrassment.

### *Exercise:*

You have noticed or suspected for some time that you're a little different from other people. You are more sensitive and you feel more deeply than others. You have difficulty separating yourself from other people's emotions. When others feel angry, hurt, or sad, it affects you deeply. You are more vulnerable to the emotional energy that surrounds you. If this is you, say, "Yep, that's me."

Speaking your truth requires that you be honest with yourself and others. Speaking your truth is difficult because it requires that you acknowledge your vulnerability. You have to learn to speak your truth to yourself first because eventually you will have to speak your truth to those who are closest to you. When you're not honest with yourself, you set yourself up to experience even more misery. You keep everything in and hide your feelings and then emotional overload hits you like a huge wave and totally engulfs you. You then slip into emotional eating, caring too much for other people's feelings and other unhealthy behaviors and habits as a way to cope with the overload of emotions.

The first step in managing your emotional overload is to speak your truth unapologetically, without shame, fear, or embarrassment. In doing this, you also learn to control your boundaries. Ever since you were young, you became easily overwhelmed by your emotions and have used food to manage your feelings. But it is time to take control of your feelings and stop allowing them to control you. Speaking your truth is liberating and empowering. All the energy you've spent hiding your emotions can be redirected in a positive way. You can love yourself for being a person who feels so deeply and at the same time look forward to learning how to manage your feelings and set boundaries for yourself.

Write the answers to the following questions in your journal and reflect on how you can speak your truth and set boundaries for yourself:

1. How have you tried to distract yourself from your feelings by eating? When was the last time you did this?
2. How has being someone who feels too much helped you in your life? In what situations has it helped you?
3. What does it feel like to have no boundaries and to let people walk all over you?
4. What would your life be like if you were able to set

boundaries and not allow people to cross those boundaries? What would you lose? How would you be different?

5. How do you try to manage your empathy for others? Are
you effective at managing your empathy toward others?

6. One person I need to set boundaries with is _____.
How will I set boundaries with them?

## DAY 22: UNDERSTANDING YOUR BOREDOM

*Food for thought:* Understanding boredom will help put an end
to the most common emotional trigger that causes overeating.

### Exercise:

Even if you're not overweight, the most common reason people overeat is out of boredom. When you're bored, the experience of eating food breaks the monotony. It typically happens
when you're watching boring TV, enjoying a lazy Sunday, studying for school, killing time, or are just bored at work. If you're
the type who always has to stay busy when you have some
downtime, you eat because you just have to be doing something. You have to fill any hole in your schedule with eating.
Understanding boredom will help put an end to this emotional
trigger that causes overeating.

Use your journal to answer the following questions:

1. Do you ever eat out of boredom?
2. How does eating when you're bored hurt you?

3. When do you find that you are most often bored? At work? Weeknights? On Sundays?

4. Do you think that you use boredom as a substitute for something? If so, for what?

5. Are there other ways you can nurture yourself and break up the monotony when you are bored? If so, what are they?

6. Are there other things that excite you besides food? If so, what are they?

## DAY 23: ENERGIZE YOUR LIFE

*Food for thought:* Watch out for people whose mere presence drains you or sucks the life out of you.

### Exercise:

Have you ever monitored your energy level and identified energizers and energy drains? When your energy falls, there is a tendency to reach for food, so keeping your energy high and balanced helps free you from emotional eating. Personal-energy work begins with monitoring your energy and discovering your energizers and drains, especially those "energy vampires."

Always beware of energy vampires, those people whose mere presence drains you or sucks the life out of you. Some people are not kind, nice, or supportive, and you should minimize or eliminate the time you spend with them. Some of us have family members or friends dampening our self-esteem every day. Even if they are your flesh and blood, try to remove yourself from their presence as much as possible. Hurtful words negate any progress toward self-worth and self-love.

In your journal, write down the names of those people, places, or things that deplete your energy. Now make a list of your Energy Pick Me-Ups, things that cause you to feel more energized. Every time you feel your energy decreasing, do one of your Energy Pick Me-Ups.

Here are some examples of Energy Pick-Me-Ups:

- *Think of something that brings you joy.* Breathe in the joy and imagine this joy moving throughout your body.
- *Stand up.* Allow your arms to make large figure-eights. Now switch and go in the other direction. As you move your arms through the air, you should feel more energized.
- *Laughter is very energizing.* Read a social media post or text from someone who makes you laugh out loud.
- *Clap your hands.* Stand and give yourself applause. Ask someone near you to do it, but if someone else can't do it for you, do it for yourself.
- *March in place*—pick up those legs as if you were doing high-knee exercises. Large-muscle movements increase the flow of energy and help you release stress.

Assess your energy right now using a 0–10 scale with 10 being the highest. If you are below a 7, do one or more of the quick-energy pick-me-ups described above or any that you've created for yourself. If your energy continues to be low, try a different energy pick-me-up until you feel more alive. Get in the habit of monitoring your energy level throughout the day and build it before it dips too low. Be aware of the energy drains so you're not blindsided by them. Remember that when your energy is low, it's easier to give in to emotional eating. The higher your energy level, the more likely you are to eat when you're actually physically hungry.

## **DAY 24:** PREPARE YOUR HOME ENVIRONMENT FOR SUCCESS

*Food for thought:* Your home environment should prepare you for success, not failure.

### *Exercise:*

Think about what your physical environment in your home looks like. Does it energize you or is it chaotic and hectic? Are there piles of clothes on the floor? Is there one room that you've been wanting to clean up? As an example, your bedroom is meant for relaxation and romance. Does your bedroom create that vibe for you? If not, maybe start there. Start small and just focus on one room that you can organize and clean up so that you will feel good to be in it. See if cleaning and organizing this one room makes you feel energized and lighter on your feet. This will also give you momentum that will allow you to clean and organize the next room. The goal is to clean up small spaces or one room or closet at a time.

Decide which room or workspace in your home you plan to

clean, organize, decorate, or liven up so that it energizes you and makes you feel good about yourself. Within the next week, focus on making that room or space a place where you will enjoy spending time.

## DAY 25: IMMERSE YOURSELF IN LEARNING

*Food for thought:* If you want to learn about or master anything in your life, you have to immerse yourself in it and let that knowledge consume you.

### Exercise:

Have you immersed yourself in learning about health and weight loss? If you want to learn about or master anything in your life, you have to immerse yourself in it. Let the knowledge consume you. I knew everything about eating clean and detoxing, which helped me stay slim. However, unexpected weight gain forced me to learn about my hormones and how they were impacting my weight. I studied over a hundred books and articles on the topic to learn everything I could about how hormones impacted weight loss, how to get tested, and what treatment options were available. I consumed information, found a hormone doctor, and successfully balanced my hormones for weight loss.

Gain knowledge of weight loss and fat burning and let this knowledge consume you. Learning about health and nutrition is where the miracle of weight loss begins. It is time to get excited about learning what will lead to greater weight-loss success. Start reading books and magazines that inspire you to eat clean, work out, or master the mental. Read success stories and other inspiring stories of weight-loss success. This will inspire you to want the same thing in your own life. Follow the footsteps of winners.

List the books, magazine, websites, or documentaries that you plan to read or study to provide you with the knowledge and inspiration to succeed on your weight-loss journey.

## DAY 26: TURN OFF YOUR TV

*Food for thought:* Know that gossip or Ratchet TV does not feed your soul or spirit.

### Exercise:

Someone once said that to be wildly successful, you have to put down the remote control and pick up a book. I took that advice to heart and it has never failed me. Give yourself a break from all television today, especially gossip or Ratchet TV, which does not feed your soul or spirit.

Also abstain from watching the news for one day. Some folks feel like they have to continuously monitor all the disasters and heartbreak in the world as if they are in charge of grief relief. See what's going on in the world, feel the feelings, take action, and then move on. You have to remember that love is still where you live, so focus on loving those in your life right now.

We have become obsessed with consuming media, from TV to social media. We wake up and check our social media accounts and television before giving any thought to God. Break that habit and seek God first thing in the morning. Don't be so eager to wake up to the things of this world. Instead, be eager to let God prepare your heart and mind for the day. Fill your life with God's presence and love.

Abstaining from idle entertainment might not be easy, but it's good for your soul. I am not telling you to do so indefinitely, but for one day you should give your mind a break from meaningless noise and chatter. No TV at all today. Instead of watching television, spend the time reading about health and nutrition. This will empower you. It's not about having someone tell you what to eat or how much to eat, that just makes you diet-minded. It's about learning how to help your unique body become healthier and lose weight. Enjoy learning, reading, and growing in knowledge. Be empowered, for knowledge is power.

## DAY 27: LEVERAGE A SUPPORT SYSTEM

*Food for thought:* Be deliberate about creating a supportive environment that can lead to long-term success.

### *Exercise:*

Don't assume a family member or friend you're closest to is the best choice for your support system. Think very deeply and be brutally honest about who has been helpful to keep you on track in the past. The best supporter will be someone who has the same goal of getting slimmer and healthier and is committed to doing whatever it takes to achieve it. It would be great if you got together to work out, do meal prep and share recipes, go grocery shopping, cook shared meals together, and if you touched base on the phone weekly. It really depends on what kind of support you actually need. Encouragement can come in many forms. Some folks just need a motivational word or quote each day to stay on track.

Also consider who is most available. Discuss how much time and energy you both have to devote to the partnership and how realistic it is to be available to support one another. Discuss what will be your primary mode of contact and support. Determine if you prefer phone, email, or text communications—this will be key to maintaining contact. If you need face-to-face time, discuss that as well and figure out the best times to get together. The goal is to ensure that there is time devoted to listening and encouraging each other.

Take a few minutes to think about what support you need on this journey. Use a journal to write down a few notes and be as specific as possible so your family members know how best to support you. An example would be, "Don't eat junk food in front of me, please go into a different room." Explicit rules will allow family members to have a better understanding of how to support you.

## DAY 28: USE A BUDDY CONTRACT

*Food for thought:* A buddy contract is the new accountability partner.

The concept of a "buddy contract" is becoming more popular in the weight-loss industry. A buddy contract is a written agreement between two or more people who commit to supporting one another on their weight-loss journey. To help ensure that both you and your support buddy get what you expect, write up a "buddy contract" that spells out your mutual goals and the ways you plan to help each other achieve them. Also, be explicit about your desired mode of communication.

The buddy contract should include both short-term goals (such as, "Meet at the gym three times a week to work out together") and long-term ones (such as, "My goal is to lose 120 pounds to achieve my ideal weight"). Just make sure the goals are specific and achievable.

Both of you should keep a copy of the agreement visibly posted somewhere so you can reread it often to remind yourself of what you're trying to accomplish.

Reevaluate your buddy relationship from time to time to ensure that it is working for both of you. Don't be afraid to call it quits when the relationship is not working out. Just like with any relationship, if you're not getting what you need, have a heart-to-heart with your buddy and either work to fix or end the buddy relationship. The purpose of the buddy relationship is to enhance the weight-loss journey for both of you and make it easier to achieve your goals.

## DAY 29: SLAY RESISTANCE IN FIVE MINUTES A DAY

*Food for thought:* A person's prayer life is a great barometer of one's spiritual health just like checking one's blood pressure is a great indicator of one's physical health.

### Exercise:

Take five minutes each day for prayer or self-reflection. You can pray or reflect on your current struggles and challenges or seek direction on what to do in any situation. I am asking you to take five minutes out of your day to make prayer and self-reflection a daily habit. Put notes up throughout your home or car until you remember this daily habit. By doing this, you are slaying resistance each day. Be aware that resistance will try to keep you from this quiet time every day. Resistance will encourage you to delay it or do it later. But take time each morning to begin your day in prayer and self-reflection.

The five-minute daily habit of prayer and self-reflection leads us to spiritual health. The more we do this, the clearer our direction becomes in our life. Five minutes a day is a simple and achievable task. Try it daily and watch your life change for the better.

## DAY 30: LIVE YOUR VERY BEST LIFE/CREATE ABUNDANCE IN YOUR LIFE

*Food for thought:* You can manifest greatness and live your full potential in every aspect of your life.

## *Exercise:*

You can visualize your perfect life and body so that you can move toward achieving those things. Begin by sitting up straight in a comfortable chair and clasp your hands loosely together in your lap. Now you want to bring awareness into your body and be present in the moment. Read the following visualization exercise out loud, and feel and embrace every word.

Imagine you have allowed greatness into every aspect of your life. Imagine you have become great and every cell in your body embodies greatness. You live a life of passion and success because you live up to your true potential. Day after day, you see life becoming healthier, happier, and more successful. You continue to see the weight melting off and you living in your ideal body. You are living a life of purpose and you see your purpose being manifested in the world. You manifest greatness and live your full potential in every aspect of life. You continue to grow and expand your knowledge and gifts. You remain on a mission and continue to fulfill your purpose.

Imagine you've mastered how to create success in every aspect of your life—spiritual, emotional, physical, financial, and professional. You are flooded with energy and have empowering success in every aspect of your life. Your success is so overflowing that it floods from your body out into the world. Your relationships at home and at work are loving and supportive. Your friendships are fun and rewarding. Your happiness and energy causes people to come up to you and ask for your help in directing them to similar success. They want to change their life because you are so amazingly successful. You are a magnet that draws people to you—they want your help with making decisions for their own life. They want the same energetic, healthy, happy life that you live. You know that for the rest of your life, you will be overflowing with abundance and be wildly successful in every aspect of your life.

You can see your energy, love, and passion for everything you wanted to be and to do in this world. You have so much light and love that everyone who sees or touches you feels it. They see your life has been transformed with amazing light, beauty, and power. You live your full potential. It manifests in so many amazing ways—health, happiness, fitness, and work. You are a light for yourself, family, and friends. You are a light in a dark world. Your beautiful light transforms everything around you. You live your highest potential of being fit, healthy, happy, smart, engaging, and loving.

## CONCLUSION

Hopefully, these exercises have established a foundation for you to create and maintain new habits to get to your goal weight and live a healthy lifestyle. I'm confident that they will help you produce long-lasting changes in yourself so that you can meet all of your health and weight-loss goals.

You can't do all exercises every single day. The goal is to do each exercise for thirty days and repeat those that are the most valuable to you.

# Part Four

---

# MOTIVATIONAL
# SUCCESS
# STORIES

Part 4, Motivational Success Stories, provides over fifteen motivational success stories and pictures of how others overcame poor eating habits, health issues, low motivation, and depression to lose the weight and keep it off. If they did it, you can too!

# 14

# Motivational Success Stories

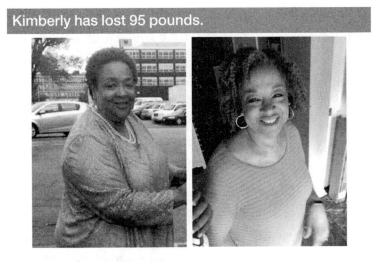

My mother suffered with morning sickness for nine months trying to bring me into this world, and when I arrived, they could not feed me fast enough! I was greedy trying to make up for lost time. As I grew up, I was fascinated with food! I learned to cook and loved to eat. Needless to say, I was a chubby kid until I played sports in high school. As I pursued higher education, I became less active, married, and started having kids of my own. My mom suffered a mild stroke at forty-eight years old. She advised me to lose weight before she passed quietly in her sleep at fifty-four years old. I was seven months pregnant with my second child at the time. Then, to my surprise, nine months later I was pregnant with our third child. I was married, with three small children and a busy career, stressed to the hilt and eating without restraint. My weight spiraled out of control as the "food-pushers" at work brought in free food from all of the best restaurants every day. I tried to ease my pain and stress with food. My heart started acting up, which was scary. I was approaching my fifth-fourth birthday, the same age my mother was when she died. It was time to get serious about my weight loss and my health. I tried every diet known to man. I even had bariatric surgery, but I always gained the weight back! Why? Because I did not change my lifestyle. I constantly went back to eating the way I always ate. You see, I knew how to cook but not how to eat! What I was feeding my body made me feel old, achy, and tired all the time.

I joined a personal training program and started working out, when someone in the group introduced us to JJ Smith and the Green Smoothie Cleanse. We tried it for ten days and I lost the most weight at 11 pounds! However, I did not know what to do to keep it going. It was not until six months later in January, that I joined JJ Smith's VIP group (a group that offers coaching by JJ Smith and long-term support for permanent weight loss) and started my first 30-Day Challenge! I lost 16 pounds and have not looked back! To date, I have lost 95 pounds! Moreover, I have kept it off. I have gone from a size 24 to a size 14. I thought my goal weight would be a size 12 but I am leaning toward a size 10. We will see!

I feel alive, energized! No need for caffeine or energy drinks. I am on fire for this new way of eating healthy, eating clean, detoxing, balancing my hormones, mastering my mind and learning how to take better care of me. My knees feel better! My blood pressure is running low and instead of taking six pills, I take just two! I broke up with diabetes; he was not the one for me. My cholesterol is normal now and my thyroid medication has been reduced! It is amazing.

I have given away my "big-girl" clothes and managed to find some hidden gems in my closet, like a fur I purchased twenty-seven years ago on my thirtieth birthday that I could never button up. I can button it up now and it fits just right! My too-little suits are now getting too big! I cannot tell you how good this feels after trying desperately for thirty years to lose weight and keep it off!

My motivation comes into full effect when I try to have a cheat meal. I think I am about to enjoy my favorite dish or snack and after a few bites, I throw it straight in the trash! My taste buds have changed and I no longer like how certain food makes my body feel—tired, sluggish, and less vibrant. The body knows! I have learned to listen and respect it.

Meal preparation is what keeps me on track. They say if you don't prepare to win, you prepare to lose! I find this to be so true when it comes to making wise choices about food. I am still a foodie at heart. I love exploring new recipes. The difference is I do not focus on what I can't or shouldn't eat. I focus on all of the new healthy things I can eat. I accept the challenge of preparing food in healthier ways without sacrificing taste!

My words of encouragement to you are to strive for progress, not perfection! Do better today than you did yesterday. That's all it takes, honestly. Remember, this is a journey not a sprint! Stay the course and you will be surprised at your results! I am the smallest I have been in over thirty years! Most of my friends have never seen me this small. JJ Smith and her team teach you how to feed your body, mind, spirit, and your wallet! She lifts you up and is so encouraging!

I am a certified GSC Leader who is trying to improve the health of folks in my neck of the woods! JJ has taught me ways to take care of the body that medical school never did. Enough said.

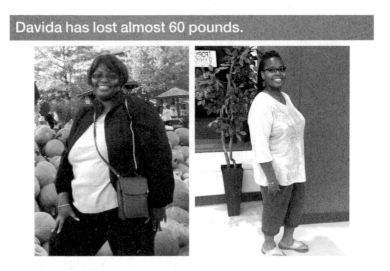

Davida has lost almost 60 pounds.

After carrying excess weight for most of my life, trying various diets and still no real success, I finally prayed on the issue. I asked God to show me what to do to have lasting success, not a quick fix. I was thumbing through Facebook, as I normally do, when I started noticing various posts on JJ Smith 10-Day

Cleanse. The before and after pictures and testimonials caught my attention and I decided to join the next group cleanse.

I began my journey on February 9th with my first full cleanse and lost 12.2 pounds that first round. My journey to my goal weight continues, but to date I have lost 58 pounds. This has definitely become a lifestyle change for me over the last two years and one that I will maintain.

For years, I suffered with high cholesterol and was prescribed cholesterol-lowering statin medication. I never liked taking any prescribed medication, especially the statin due to the side effects. In the nineteen months after I started with JJ's program, however, my doctor was so thrilled with my weight loss (my vitals came back in a healthy range) that I was taken off the cholesterol medication. My iron levels also improved to an acceptable range. As I regularly say, "Green Smoothies do the body good." Not only has my health improved but also my skin is glowing. I feel more youthful than I had previously felt in many years.

My family has been my greatest motivation, especially my mother. She has a heart of gold, but unfortunately suffers with numerous health challenges, some of which could improve with dietary changes and weight loss. She encourages me to press on and continue to take care of my health, because it is hard to get back once you lose it. I want to change the face of the generational curses that have plagued my extended family for far too long. I am thankful to be such an inspiration to my family and friends. Many have told me that I inspire them to press on, exercise, and eat healthier options. To God be the glory. We can walk by faith, but faith without works (healthier food choices and exercise) is dead.

To remain motivated, I stay close to JJ's Facebook group for inspiration and support. I meal-plan, shop, and prep for the week. I also keep healthy snacks on hand at all times to ward off hunger. I would advise anyone on this journey to believe in yourself and tell yourself daily . . . "I got this!"

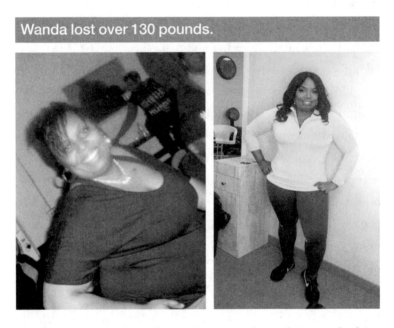

Wanda lost over 130 pounds.

My name is Wanda Belizario. I remember when my highest point ironically became the lowest point in my life. Being 5'6" and reaching an all-time high weight of 342 pounds destroyed what little self-esteem I had left after being in an abusive relationship for two years, then a silent emotional one for several years. That is truly when, unbeknownst to me, I had internally lost myself and tried to hide my depression under food. Because I allowed myself to believe that I was smaller than what I was, to the outside world I looked happy. This worked great for some time. I hid under big T-shirts, wore sweatpants, and always had my clothes tailored—not wanting to know my actual size. I was selective with whom I shared vacation pictures and I was mostly always covered with a towel embarrassed about how I looked in a swimsuit. Then there was the development of social media.

Little did I know that social media, which I initially feared because of the pressure to post pictures and videos, would become my salvation. While I had control over what I posted, I had no control over the pictures posted of me by someone else. I remember one post that did it for me, it was like being forced to look at myself and the comments of shock and disbelief from people who had not seen me in years. It killed me. I felt crushed. Yet it was then that I decided to do something about it. First, I visited my doctor who recommended I see a nutritionist. The nutritionist suggested that I start slow, reducing daily calories, not to expect things to happen fast and to make sure I was mentally ready for the change.

Searching the Internet, I found a video of this woman who stated I could lose up to 10 pounds without going to the gym. I was so happy because the gym was one place I did not want to go; I then made a purchase that would change my life forever. I bought JJ Smith's book *The 10-Day Green Smoothie Cleanse* and actually read it in one day, while I admittedly ate several snacks. I talked to people at work in search of someone to try the cleanse with me and one friend agreed. Every other form of support came from the JJ Smith Green Smoothie Cleanse Facebook page. The encouragement there was so motivating and spirit-raising, I felt a great connection. I couldn't wait to post the pic of my veggies, fruits, snacks, and new Nutribullet I purchased. I was so excited to post.

I knew then this was going to work. Even though I had said it many times before, this time I felt it in my heart. Being a virgin to detoxing, I messed up in the first three days of my 10-day cleanse. Yet the encouragement from JJ Smith herself on the page and others truly helped motivate me and align my will-power with my goal. I restarted my ten days and successfully finished. I was amazed at how good I felt, amazed at my ability to not eat rice, platano, salami or to drink coffee. Being a Dominican woman, that was hard for me. Then it happened—the biggest payoff to my sacrifice—getting on the scale and seeing I was 12 pounds lighter! The excitement I felt was heard throughout the building in which I live. It was then that I thought to myself, "You did this without exercising, girl. Go see what happens when you go to the gym." That began my next twice-a-month 10-Day Green Smoothie Cleanse, along with the gym, for the next two years.

While signing up at the local YMCA, this one question on the paperwork made me think of JJ Smith. The question asked, "What motivated me to begin my membership?" Immediately, I smiled and thought of JJ Smith! She tricked me into positivity. She knew that after seeing the weight loss I would be motivated to push further and want to work out. JJ Smith also motivated me to challenge myself, and I joined something I was always afraid of, an intense boot camp workout program. With the combination of all three, especially the 10-Day Green Smoothie Cleanse, the pounds really started to shed. My results even encouraged family members and coworkers to try the Green Smoothie Cleanse and it has been successful for them as well.

I never thought that the sad 342-pound me that began my 10-Day Green Smoothie Cleanse journey in 2014 would ever see a spiritually better 210-pound me with more self-esteem. JJ Smith's method of cleaning my body has taught me how to eat right and healthy. Her dedication to us through her videos and Facebook page maintains my motivation. I'm truly living now because I'm happy inside and out, no more faking it. Instead of beating myself up, I know how to get back on track if I mess up. I vacation more, have more energy, and encourage others. I am finally the total me I knew and always wanted to be. I am happy and living in my "You Only Live Once" moment to the fullest.

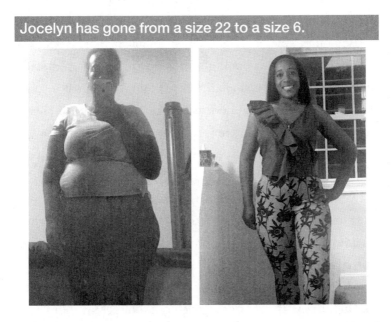

Jocelyn has gone from a size 22 to a size 6.

It was December and I was at my breaking point. I suffered from inflammation, bloating, slow metabolism, foggy brain, and severe back and knee pain. In the month of February, I gave birth to a beautiful, healthy baby girl! However, during my pregnancy, I worried about weight gain because I was already tipping the scale at 214 pounds. I gained 20 pounds during pregnancy, I lost 20 pounds after I gave birth, and then gained the 20 pounds right back! Frustrated, weighing in at 234 pounds, I joined JJ's VIP group and my life has never been the same.

I have lost 75 pounds in less than a year and dropped from a size 22 dress to a size 6!

My self-image has improved, my energy has increased, I have a clearer mind, there is no bloating or inflammation, and I'm happy to say my back and knee pain are gone!

What keeps me inspired and motivated every day is prayer and devotion, starting my day with this portion keeps my mind focused on the blessings that I've been given. Secondly, sticking close to the Facebook group keeps my mind connected with others who have similar goals. JJ Smith is a great teacher and when I practice the information that she teaches I always have success. Lastly, I am now a mother of a beautiful baby girl and I want to be a positive example to teach her how to avoid obesity and other health risks.

A few strategies that I have learned to use are to set long, short, intermittent, and daily goals. I also reward myself when I achieve my goals, which keeps me motivated during the journey.

My mind-set is such that when setbacks arise, I never give up. On the days that I want to give up, I redirect my mind back to my planned goals. Support. Support. Support. I attempted to rid unwanted pounds many times, but without proper support it was an epic fail. So, get the support you need to be successful on this weight-loss journey.

**Michelle has lost over 60 pounds.**

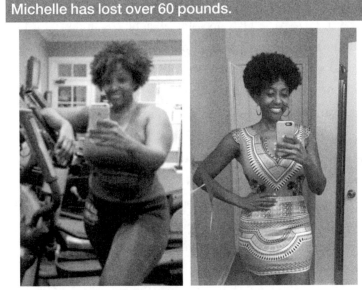

I am forty-five years old and my "get optimally healthy" journey started in January. At that time, I made a commitment to myself to become the most disciplined person I know. I was determined to totally reverse the outcome of my health assessment, which was done in mid-December. I weighed in at 224 pounds, had high blood pressure, high cholesterol and felt plain miserable. Something about those red exclamation marks on a piece of paper ignited a flame in me and started me on my way. I knew I had two choices: do nothing and allow my health to further deteriorate *or* do something to steer totally away from "danger zone." Through grace and mercy, I chose the latter.

In January, I started researching anything and everything I could that had to do with losing weight and improving my health overall (mind, body, and soul). Then came JJ Smith and the world-renowned green smoothies. After extensive research, I added green smoothies to my daily regimen. I told myself at the very beginning that I would not rush the process, as I wanted to MASTER my mind, weight loss, and weight-loss maintenance for good! By the time my health assessment rolled around a year later, I was down 50 pounds and vital statistics were "normal." The nurse who completed my assessment gave me a "gold star" for reversing my prior year's results!

As a result of dropping the 50 pounds, my abnormal breathing pattern returned to normal. Also, my digestive system, which was at the brink of a shutdown, began to function properly again. I was so ecstatic about my results that I challenged myself to drop another 14 pounds just for general purpose. Four months later I was down to 160 pounds for a total weight loss of 64 pounds.

To stay motivated, I *always* keep the reason why I started my journey at the forefront of my mind. Frankly, I've come too far to turn back now. My family and I deserve the improved healthier version of myself. Also, I challenge myself on a constant and consistent basis to keep improving without stopping. "Me vs. me, I will not lose" is the motto that I live by.

The one thing I would advise anyone who is on the journey is to feed their mind with as much positivity as they possibly can on a daily basis. It takes a healthy *mind* to obtain and sustain a healthy lifestyle.

Carol has lost 70 pounds.

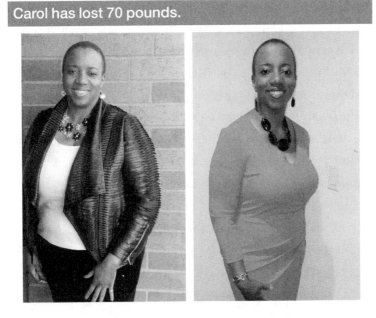

I began my journey in January. As a child, I was raised in a home with a lot of love. There was love everywhere, but as you know, unless you truly love yourself, there is something missing. Deep down I didn't love myself as I should have. Years and years and years of disappointment, being self-conscious, upset, and not loving the skin that I was in had come to a head. I tried every diet known to man yet over the years, I kept getting bigger and bigger. When I stepped on the scale and I saw 237 pounds and I was wearing a size 20/22, I'd had it. Diabetes, high blood pressure, high cholesterol, and heart disease ran in my family. I already had high blood pressure and high cholesterol and was headed on a freight train toward diabetes and heart disease. I had to do something about it. I saw information on Facebook about a 30-Day Challenge that JJ Smith was going to have. I thought to myself, "Carol, this is your time." I prepared myself mentally to begin right after I returned home from vacation. I knew I was going to start a few days late, but I had to start in order to save my life.

My lifestyle change consisted of having two smoothies a day and one clean meal along with healthy snacks. I began exercising three to four times a week and I loved it. I increased it to five-six times a week on some weeks. Part of the DHEMM (Detox/Hormonal Balance/Eat Clean/Mental Mastery/Move) system is to Move. I found that moving helped me as much mentally as it did physically. The inches and the weight just began to fall off. I made sure that I stayed hydrated by drinking half my body weight in ounces of water. That was key to my success because it helped flush the toxins that had built up in my body. I finally got my mind right. I was able to be really focused, in spite of all that was going on in the world around me. Yes, there are still stresses in my life and ups and downs, but I handle things differently with the education and knowledge that I have gained from JJ Smith, the ambassadors, and the VIP group.

I am so happy and proud to say that I have lost 70 pounds and am a size 10/12. I walk with a pep in my step and have gotten both my sexy and my confidence back. The doctor ran tests and all of my numbers are better. I am now off my blood pressure medication. I continue to drink my water and exercise. I travel a lot for work, so I may not exercise as much some months, but I have still been able to maintain my weight loss. I equip myself with the tools that I need to succeed while I am away from home for extended periods of time. I still make my smoothies every morning, I prepare my snacks, and I plan ahead.

I am motivated to be around to see my nieces and nephews graduate, go to college, get married, and have kids. I did not want to be the Auntie that passed away at an early age due to obesity and all of the health issues that came along with it.

If there is one thing that I can tell you as you are reading my segment in this book, it is to never give up on yourself. You have the inner strength to be the best you that you can be. Just take it one day at a time, literally. Plan for tomorrow and then when that day is done, plan for the next tomorrow and then the next. Before you know it, you will be a much healthier and most likely a much happier you. Love yourself enough to take that first step.

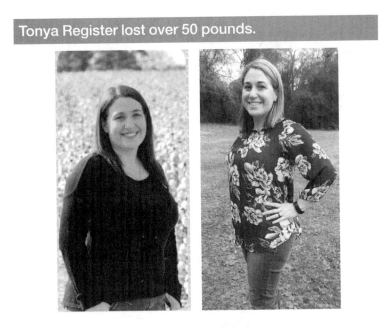

Tonya Register lost over 50 pounds.

I started my journey a little over two years ago with at 10-day cleanse and had great success losing 20 pounds in ten days. I then signed up to be a VIP member and I participated in JJ's Flat Belly Challenge. I did have some success, but not the results I wanted because I still had not fully committed to my weight-loss journey. At that time, I had several distractions in my life. I was enrolled in my master's classes for science of nursing. I found myself divorced and back to being a single momma of five children. Needless to say, my weight-loss journey took a back seat to everything else I had going on. In 2017, I started the year off by marrying my best friend and biggest supporter. After seeing myself in our wedding pictures, I knew I needed to do something. I would do a full cleanse, lose weight and stick to it for a little while before I would go back to eating the same way I had before, putting all of the weight back on.

I would watch people in the VIP group post about their weight loss and feel guilty because I knew that I could do that too. In November, I got serious about my weight loss. I weighed 198 pounds and had a waist that measured 43 inches. I have a watched my mother and aunts struggle with their weight my entire life and I did not want to do the same thing. Plus, I wanted to be healthy for my children. I wanted energy to play with my toddler and to look good so that I did not embarrass my older children. I did a 10-day full cleanse before Thanksgiving and, of course, everyone thought I was crazy. I heard it all from "Are you drinking sewage water?" to "I couldn't drink that, it looks horrible?" These same people now ask me what I have done to lose all my weight. I tell people that this lifestyle is easy because I don't have to count calories or macros of any kind. I eat clean and my body loves it. I did the Killer Curves Challenge this year, a challenge where you focus on losing the weight, but keeping your curves. My waist was 41 inches at the start of it, and as of this writing, my waist measures 27 inches. I am down to 146 pounds and my goal is 138. I have learned to drink my water everyday and I've come to understand how detoxing the body does help with weight loss. I have taken what I learned and am currently helping my husband and son lose weight. I convinced my husband to have his hormones checked because he carries a lot of his weight in his stomach area. Initially, he argued with me that everything was okay. I knew better—imagine his surprise when I was right. He is now getting hormone therapy and I am sure that he will start losing weight too.

This is a lifestyle not a diet. It has completely changed my life and I feel better now than I did when I was in my twenties. I can talk for hours about JJ and the green smoothies because they literally saved me from being overweight and miserable. I try to encourage everyone who is on a weight-loss journey to be consistent and drink their water. I am truly living my best life!

**Kortni has lost 50 pounds.**

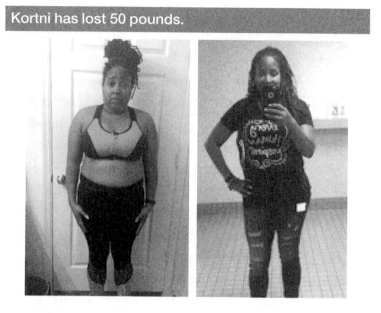

I started my weight-loss journey in September. I traveled home for a visit, and while I was there, I had to switch from my loose and flowing maxi dresses and actually put on clothes. It was then that I realized my jeans and shirts were tight! And, of course, when you're visiting your peeps, you want to take pictures. I guess before that I had not been taking that many pictures. Needless to say, it was not a pretty sight.

While home, I was talking to my bestie's sister, Marcia, and she told me how she too was about to get on the ball and take control of her weight. She'd heard about the 10-Day Green Smoothie Cleanse and had been gifted a book. I told her I had lost weight doing smoothies before too and planned to go back to replacing one meal a day with a smoothie. I lost both my father and mother to cancer and did not want that to be my story. I went back home and started going to the gym and having a smoothie for breakfast (only I was not making them the correct way, aka the green way).

Six months later, I was 17 pounds lighter, and I saw a picture of Marcia. She looked FABULOUS!! I immediately asked what she was doing, and she reminded me that she was doing the green smoothies. She had first started with the 10-day cleanse and had moved on to the Green Smoothies for Life. I committed right then and there.

In March of last year my life changed. I embarked on the Green Smoothie lifestyle, and have not turned back since. Prior to that, I was constantly plagued by sinus infections, diagnosed with sinusitis. I had horrible allergies and was doing immunotherapy shots (two shots, twice per week for twelve weeks before I was able to reach a monthly dosage) along with taking Zyrtec and Claritin every day. I also had severe acid reflux, IBS, and was prone to migraines. When I started the 10-day cleanse, I immediately noticed a change. I was not having the ice-pick migraines; I was not constantly draining in the back of my throat, and I had more energy.

I could go on all day about the benefits I have reaped on the Green Smoothie lifestyle, but I have limited space! I have been living the Green Smoothie lifestyle for six months now and have lost a total of 50 pounds and numerous inches. I can honestly tell you what keeps me going on my journey is the ease of what I am doing. If I do not have a Green Smoothie, I am missing it and my body is craving one. And the best part: I feel as if I am eating and snacking more now than when I was eating and drinking whatever I wanted.

I no longer crave the junk food. I'm never hungry and always satisfied. Yet, I am continuing to lose weight and inches! Who does that? I do, with the help and support of JJ and the 10-Day Green Smoothie Cleanse crew. My skin is clear and glowing and I feel as good as I look. I would tell anyone who is thinking about embarking on this lifestyle, the key to being successful is to detox!

When I tell you JJ Smith is the truth, she is the truth! She doesn't just help you lose the weight by giving you recipes to follow. JJ helps you break the chains of food addiction! The Detox/Hormonal Balance/Eat Clean/Mental Mastery/Move System is my life, and something that has allowed me to attain what I've been trying to do all of my life: manage my weight and be healthy.

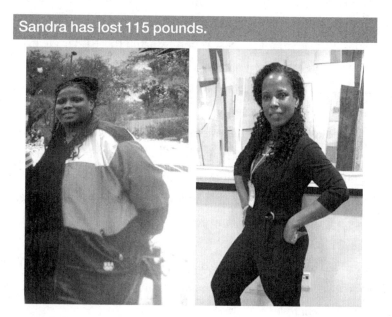

Sandra has lost 115 pounds.

I began my weight-loss journey in April, weighing in at 277 pounds. I heard about the 10-Day Green Smoothie Cleanse and began doing research on it for about three weeks. I joined the 10-Day Green Smoothie Cleanse Facebook page and read all of the testimonials. I saw other people having success on this program and I thought to myself: "Wow, Sandra, that could be you one day!" For years I had tried to lose weight. I made some progress but nothing really significant. I finally made up my mind to give this 10-Day Green Smoothie Cleanse a try, and boy, am I glad I did. This cleanse totally changed and transformed my life. I have lost a total of 115 pounds. I have gone from a size 22/24 to a size 4/6/8!

I started because I knew there had to be more in life. I wanted more, more energy, the glowing skin, more mobility. I wanted to be around to see and help raise my grandchildren. When more becomes your objective, less becomes unacceptable. I wanted and needed to make a change. With discipline, dedication, determination, and a made-up mind, I did just that! I took a leap and I have never regretted it.

The health conditions that have improved: I now have more energy. People are constantly telling me that I need to slow down; I merely look them in the eye and tell them they need to catch up! My skin used to itch from me being so toxic, but as a result of implementing daily detox methods, I no longer have that issue because my skin absolutely glows. And all of this was done naturally. No surgery. Just detoxing, becoming aware of my hormone imbalances, eating clean and healthy, mastering my mental well-being, and moving daily.

My "why" is my motivation. I remember why I started. I remember how I used to feel prior to the 10-day cleanse. Severely overweight and unhealthy, I was lethargic and inactive. I was bloated and unhappy. I did not like what I saw when I looked in the mirror. I was simply tired of looking and feeling the way I did. Later I joined the VIP group, and the support and accountability I discovered became a lifeline for me. Now in a sisterhood of love and acceptance, I was able to reach out to like-minded individuals. Everyone understood the journey. We may have been at different places on our journey but our destination was the same. Advancing from the 10-Day Green Smoothie Cleanse to the incorporation of the DHEMM System (Detox/Hormonal Balance/Eat Clean/Mental Mastery/Move), I was able to maximize my weight-loss results. Optimal health was and is still the ultimate goal!

Weight loss will come eventually but the scale will not determine how we view ourselves. My motivation is to remind myself of what God has done and will continue to do in my life. I must do the work, results will come. Without challenge, there is no change!

The one thing I would say to inspire someone else on their weight-loss journey is to stay the course. Do not quit! Yes, you may stumble; you may even fall, but you simply must not quit . . . Implement my DARE system into your life.

**D:** *Dream It!* Dream the size/weight you want to be. See it in your mind.

**A:** *Aim for It!* Do what you must to get there (eat clean, move, detox, balance your hormones, mental mastery).

**R:** *Reach it!* No matter how long it takes, reach your desired goal! It may take one year, two years, or even three, but reach it!

Then

**E:** *Excel at it!* That's right, excel at your new lifestyle! Master this craft of losing weight and keeping it off! Read JJ's books and join the VIP group!! Do whatever it takes to excel! DARE to do it.

This journey has saved my life. It is one I embrace daily and celebrate annually. I know the day I was born. I do not know the day I will leave this earthly home but I know the day my life changed for the better. The day I did my first 10-day cleanse!

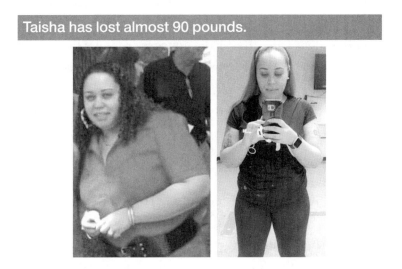

Taisha has lost almost 90 pounds.

My name is Taisha Young and I decided to begin my weight-loss/health journey about two years ago. Before I made this life-changing decision, I was in a very dark place in my life. Severely depressed, I had no confidence and no motivation. Smiling on the outside, I was crying on the inside. I sheltered myself. I hated who I'd become and had almost lost everything I owned.

I was only twenty-seven years old when all of the above caused me to be on seventeen different medications. Yes, seventeen! I had very high blood pressure, migraines, suffered memory loss (literally writing everything on sticky notes), and my anxiety was through the roof. I eventually had a stroke and a mild heart attack! For almost two months, I was literally in the ER two to three days every week! I thought I was dying. It was the most terrifying experience that has happened in my life.

It was my family and my boyfriend who told me they were worried about my health and desired for me to get healthy again. They knew I was depressed, and we all know depression is a silent killer. It was the concern from my loved ones that made me want to become motivated again. I made them a promise that I would take better care of myself. Not only that, my two boys needed their goofy and happy mother back. I really hated for my kids to see me in this position and experience the energy I was giving off. I began to change my thought process immediately. I weighed the most I have ever weighed in my life at 250 pounds! I am only 5'1". At this time, I was twenty-eight years old. I could drink two 2-liter sodas a day and eat an entire large pepperoni pizza by myself. I remember watching Steve Harvey's talk show one day; he had JJ Smith as a guest to talk about her *10-Day Green Smoothie Cleanse* book. She immediately grabbed my attention with her confidence, how healthy she looked, and her glowing skin. Her lifestyle change gave me the motivation I needed. I immediately downloaded her book on my phone, went to the grocery store and bought everything I needed to begin this lifestyle change.

I remember reading a quote, "When you become lazy, it's disrespectful to those who believe in you." Those words spoke volumes to me. I stopped drinking sodas cold turkey. I threw away all of my medication and switched them out for vitamins instead. I no longer buy unhealthy snacks, juices, et cetera; only water and almond milk. I was suspicious about trying out the green smoothies, but they taste really good. The first two days, I was starving. I made a smoothie for breakfast and one for lunch. I ate healthy snacks in between meals, drank lots of water to keep me full and for dinner, I would eat a small-portioned healthy meal. By day 6, I felt alive! My energy was up, I did not feel tired or lazy, and I felt a difference in my weight already. I stepped on the scale to weigh myself and discovered I was already down 14 pounds! My skin began clearing up and I was able to think clearly again. After my 10-day detox ended, I continued to make a green smoothie for breakfast every morning. I drank a gallon of water a day with a few lemon slices in it. I completely cut out fried foods, pork, beef, and sodas. I mostly ate (besides the green smoothies) turkey, chicken, and fish. I walked a mile a day in my neighborhood and would keep moving so as not to become lazy. The most important factor was getting plenty of rest.

In six months, I was already down 73 pounds! I am currently thirty years old and am proud of myself for beginning a journey that changed my lifestyle. To be honest, it was not easy, but I kept my faith through it all. Take it one day at a time. Do not think about tomorrow or next week, you're already getting ahead of yourself. Excuses are not motivational. Love yourself and take care of yourself first and foremost, then everything else will fall into place. I gained my confidence back (plus more), I'm genuinely smiling, full of energy, no longer lazy, and above all, I'm healthy. I still have bad days as well, but even through those days I try to stay positive. If there was any advice I could give, it would be to believe in yourself. Be the role model you would want your kids to look up to, never feed into negative energy (you will have people who will doubt you), focus on self-growth. You never know who you will inspire or who looks up to you. Put yourself and your NEEDS first.

I currently weigh 163 pounds, I am down 87 pounds. I'm still not where I want to be, but I'm working on it and still drinking my green smoothies. Also, I am no longer having health issues.

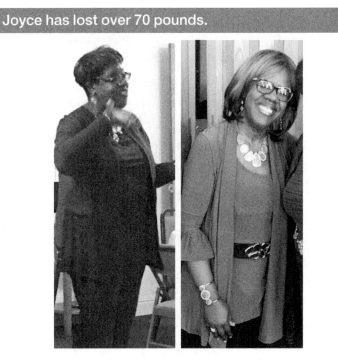

Joyce has lost over 70 pounds.

I thought that I had finally made progress with my "baby weight" ten years ago. I was back in a size 8. Then, I found myself in a spiral of life-altering events. I was diagnosed with breast cancer (my sister was diagnosed two months earlier). Less than two months after completion of my nine-month treatment, my mother was diagnosed with terminal cancer. I became one of her caregivers. A month after her passing, my daughter moved away to attend college, my job relocated (after twenty-seven years), and I entered a PhD program. I managed to lose 30 pounds in 2014, to a size 16, in preparation for my twenty-five-year vow renewal. However, I soon lost control again and packed on weight when I started teleworking three days a week while balancing family life, school, and health/caregiving issues with my dad and husband.

I attended the graduation for my PhD in Florida in January. To celebrate, my husband and I tacked on a cruise to the Bahamas and did a mini-hike while on the trip. As I trekked down a slope, I slipped and fell. It was not until we were on our plane ride home that I started to feel the effects. By the time we arrived home, I could barely walk. I went to the doctor and learned that I had bilateral osteoarthritis, severe in one knee. One of the doctor's recommendations was to lose weight to take stress off the joints. I had to do something. I owned a copy of *10-Day Green Smoothie Cleanse* and started with a 10-day modified cleanse in early February. I lost 8 pounds. I then bought the 30-Day Program, *Green Smoothies for Life*. Upon completion of the 30-Day Program, I learned of the VIP group. I wanted to be at my goal weight (the weight I was when I was diagnosed) at my ten-year cancerversary. I joined the VIP group and have lost over 55 pounds since beginning my #GS4L (Green Smoothies for Life) journey. I am closing in on my 72-pound goal.

At age fifty-seven, a number of changes have taken place in my body. Good nutrition to support health and regular physical activity to maintain mobility is even more important now.

God has a plan! He wants us to be healthy, well, and fit. Our bodies are the temple of the Holy Ghost. As good stewards, we have a responsibility to take good care of our bodies, including the basics, like eating well, sleeping well, and getting enough exercise. Even amidst our frailties, God sees the desires of our hearts. He helps and encourages us through the power of the Holy Spirit and His Word. He is the Ultimate Motivator. "Delight thyself also in the Lord. And He shall give you the desires of thine heart." (Psalms 37:4) Being part of a supportive community, JJ Smith's Private VIP Group, makes all the difference in the world. My self-determination is strong, but I also need to be encouraged and held accountable. Also, the tips and challenges from the group keep motivation high. And, detoxing is a game-changer.

One tip that I would share with others on this health and weight-loss journey is this easy and effective way to incorporate activity into your day. For years when I worked on-site, I walked during my breaks and for fifteen minutes of my lunch hour to maintain my weight. Now that I am teleworking, I use my Fitbit to monitor my steps as I step in place with hand weights during breaks and fifteen minutes of my lunch. I put on a recorded television show so that I'm not bored. Do what works for you and that which you can do consistently.

Just as GS4L is a not a diet but a lifestyle, good health is a journey not a destination!

Bolesha has maintained her 70-pound weight loss.

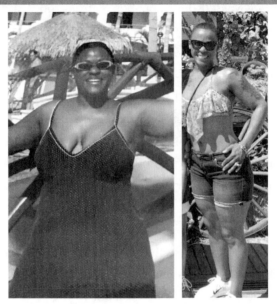

I got serious about my health when I was diagnosed with Crohn's disease and Sarcoid. I felt my body was deteriorating. Both of these conditions are stress-induced. In my career, I supervise administrators who impact the lives of children and families that have been involved with child-abuse cases. Learning of my condition was a true wake-up call. The physician was very condescending when delivering my medical options. While driving home, I vividly recall the feeling of powerlessness.

That is when I decided to change my life and take the power back over my life. I joined a gym and started to monitor my food. I was able to lose approximately 50 pounds and maintain that for several years. I was pleased with my progress, but I felt my weight loss was stagnant. I then learned about the Green Smoothie Cleanse and it changed my life forever. I learned the importance of detoxing and how it contributes to weight loss. This was an awakening for me. I took full advantage of the VIP privileges and studied all the information JJ provided. She explains things so simply. I was so impressed with the shared knowledge, I became an affiliate and opened my business, Fit, Fine & Fabulous. I clearly understand how various foods affect my body. My determination and commitment to my health has contributed to lasting results. I feel in control and empowered. I have maintained a weight loss of 70 pounds.

I truly believe I can achieve anything I desire. I have created success over the course of my life and now the benefits are abundant. I love how I feel and look. Every day, I get a choice to choose the life I want.

- I choose to have that relationship.
- I choose to respond to that circumstance.
- I choose to allow this and that to affect me negatively.

I am in a place, as I turn fifty years old, where I believe that I deserve the best the world has to offer. I'm happy, content, confident, discerning, and focused on what God has for me. I have done my work to get to this place and now I want to give back. I am now obtaining my life-coaching certificate to help others move their lives forward.

My final advice: You can do anything you put your mind to. First, believe you're worthy of the change and make active efforts to achieve your goal, then celebrate. Purposely set up small achievements, this builds confidence, motivation, and success. You cannot take on another person's decision. Everyone has to take control of their own life.

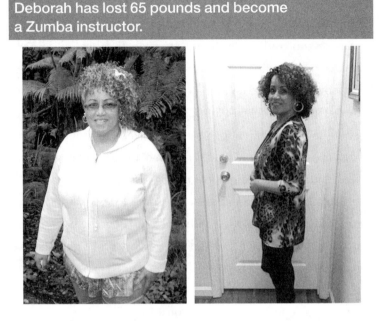

Deborah has lost 65 pounds and become a Zumba instructor.

In October I experienced acute pain across my lower back and immediately left work to go to the emergency room. I thought it was kidney stones, based on experience, so I was not prepared for the diagnosis of diverticulitis (inflamed intestines). The emergency doctor administered an intensive antibiotic. He also explained that once this condition appears, it *will* recur. Since I did not receive any advice or guidance on how to deal with this condition other than see my primary physician, I did my research via the internet, which ultimately led me to JJ's book *Lose Weight Without Dieting or Working Out!* To my horror, I learned that I had done this to myself by:

1. *Not taking my health conditions seriously:* For example, I should have asked more questions of the colonoscopy doctor who examined me three years earlier

to determine if I was a candidate for this condition and what I could do to prevent it. I did not know!

2. *Not eating the right foods:* Fruits and vegetables were missing from my daily diet. I ate fast food more days of the week than I prepared a home-cooked meal. I was a meat and potatoes person. I planned all of my meals around what meat I was eating and multiple selections of starches were always on the table. Of course, there were always a variety of desserts finding their way onto my plate.

3. *Drinking the wrong liquids:* Sodas, sweet teas, and fruit juices were my downfall. I did not drink enough water. McDonald's was one of my fast-food stops and I loved their sweet tea.

Most importantly, I learned that some of the bad health conditions that had already taken most of my senior family members and my brother were a direct result of bad eating habits. A family history of high blood pressure, strokes, diabetes, high cholesterol, sinus infections, allergies, shortness of breath, kidney problems that led to daily dialysis requirements, and obesity were starting to manifest in me.

All of this research hit me. I'm sixty-three years old, I've worked hard for others all of my life and I'm also working hard on an "accelerated path to death." I made my decision to use the advice in JJ's book to develop a healthy lifestyle plan for me. A plan that focused on eating healthier, enjoying life, and seeing if I could lose weight without working out. I had not exercised in over twenty-three years and I knew I wasn't ready to incorporate that into my plan. Special note: I already had JJ's book, I'd skimmed through it but I had not incorporated the information into my life. Something has to occur in your life to make you want to change.

I reached my goal of improved health and a surprising weight loss just six months after starting JJ's Green Smoothie Modified Cleanse, which I have maintained with weight fluctuations of up to 10 pounds for three years. During this time, I've incorporated JJ's DHEMM program and continue having at least one green smoothie on most days. I monitor my weight fluctuations and make corrections in what I'm eating and doing to get back on my plan. Two years ago, I started various types of exercise classes. I enjoyed the music and socialization so much that I made a plan to acquire my Zumba license within a year. I reached that goal and started applying for positions. I was hired to hold my first class within five months. I never imagined that at sixty-seven years old, I would be alive and a Zumba instructor. Tears come to my eyes when I think of the value of JJ's guidance and how much she has given of herself to help us live.

I know I was over 200 pounds, but I didn't know my exact weight because I was too afraid of getting on the scale; I never wanted to see that number. I did not weigh myself until I was over my diverticulitis and had already changed what I was eating. The scale read 198 pounds and I can only imagine what I weighed originally. I tracked my weight loss based on that lower scale reading; I've lost 65 pounds and a lot of inches. I was wearing sizes XL and 18. Now I'm wearing XS/S and 4/6, depending on the garment style. This outcome was a surprise for me since my original goal was to be able to wear the clothes in size 12/14 that were in my closet. I had to reset my goals based on what was best for my body.

My cholesterol level has dropped from 212 and I'm maintaining at 125–132. My pre-diabetes condition is gone. I no longer need my asthma and inflammation-reduction medications. I have more energy whereas before I constantly needed to sit down since I was frequently out of breath with a racing heart. I have not had a recurrence of inflamed bowels (diverticulitis).

My fuzzy-brain feeling and lack of clear thinking for concentration is gone.

I stay inspired with the help of God, my family, and JJ's Facebook forums, activities, and calls, which allowed me to learn from others' testimonies and learn about new "tools" to incorporate into my healthy lifestyle plan. This inspires me to reach out to others and help them learn how they can also live healthier lives.

I never want to experience diverticulitis again. Due to inflamed intestines, I was in excruciating pain, bloated, miserable, and I did not have a bowel movement for over ten days.

I think about being around as long as I can to have the energy to hang out with my granddaughters. I want to actively be able to do what they do. Nothing gives me more joy than seeing the little ones' faces when I climb and run around on the playground equipment with them and slide down the sliding boards.

I love the feeling of putting on an outfit, which I could not even have imagined getting into, and finding that not only does it fit but it looks good and feels good.

I want to grow up gracefully and extend my quality of life for as long as I can. At the same time, I love extending God's love through a smile, a hug, encouragement, inspiration, and acts of kindness to others.

I want to be a walking testimony to my family that we can overcome our family's medical history of bad health.

If a sixty-three-year-old, post-menopausal woman who did not exercise can do this, you can do this! Focus on eating to be healthy and the weight loss will be a fantastic outcome. Plan, shop, and prepare your meals so that you are not hungry and searching for food. Find ways to have fun and enjoy life that do not center on food. As JJ says, "Food does not equal fun."

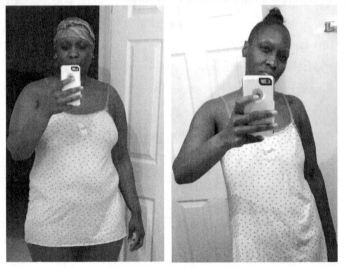

Elaine has lost almost 70 pounds.

I started this weight-loss journey 18 months ago. I awoke one morning, looked in the mirror, and discovered I had gained 60 pounds. I did not like the image I saw in the mirror and no longer wanted my husband to see me with all of the extra weight. I hated the way my body appeared before me, and no longer looked like the woman he originally married.

I have lost a total of 67 pounds and feel great! I no longer suffer from constant fatigue and now have energy to work out daily. What keeps me inspired and motivated is checking in on JJ Smith's online VIP daily and sharing my weight-loss story with anyone and everyone I can. I have inspired my sister, her friend, and a few of my friends to join the "Green Smoothie Life." Knowing that they are watching my progress holds me accountable for my actions, and as a result, I have managed to keep the weight off for a year now!

One strategy I use to stay motivated is allowing myself to have one or two cheat meals per week. Since I eat clean all week long, the cheat meal gives me something to look forward to, considering I'm not really a health guru.

The one thing I would say to encourage someone to continue on this health and weight-loss journey is that I did not think I was going to last two days, but I did and I promise you it does get easier with each passing day. It becomes a way of life, a habit, so to speak.

You may encounter a few setbacks. It is okay, just get right back on it. You are going to have better health, more energy, and when you look in that mirror you are going to love the image that is looking back at you. It's so worth it.

Girosalee has lost 60 pounds.

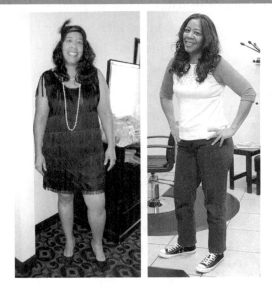

I started the Green Smoothie Cleanse two years ago. I tried so many different diets, from the Atkins diet to the Cardiac diet to Weight Watchers. All of these were a temporary solution to my weight loss. After almost giving up, having two children, and going through a divorce, I found JJ Smith. I contacted her through Facebook messenger to ask her about her program. She told me about the program and that I needed the book to get started. She also informed me about the VIP group, which helps you hold yourself accountable and get support from thousands of others on the same journey. I purchased the book, joined the VIP group, and was determined to not make excuses for the weight that I was holding on to. Since committing to this journey, I have lost 60 pounds, going from a size 22/24 to a 12/14. I have not looked back.

I never thought of myself as a big person, but I did find myself unhappy. I always tried to stay active to keep up with my children. However, my knees and back would ache when I tried to run with them. I was always tired and needed to take naps throughout the day. When I first started the journey, I could see the yellow in my eyes and acne on my face and arms that I wanted to get rid of. It was not a hard decision to believe that a program with ingredients that were natural could help heal my body. I had nothing to lose, just opportunities to gain.

After completing the 10-Day Green Smoothie Cleanse, I had so much energy, my face started to clear up, and my knees didn't ache as much. JJ says listen to your body, so I did as much as I could to "move," and the weight just kept coming off. I received compliments at work, many questions about how I did it, and I even had men approaching me. Buying a new wardrobe was not disappointing. I lost 50 pounds in five months by following the 10-Day Green Smoothie Cleanse, adding exercise to my daily routine, and living the DHEMM (Detox/Hormonal Balance/Eat Clean/Mental Mastery/Move) lifestyle. My knees and back no longer hurt and I have that "Green Smoothie glow."

A few tips I would encourage anyone on this journey to embrace are to make drinking half of your body weight in water a goal. Make sure to eat every two to three hours to keep triggering your metabolism and find some way to move. I do have an accountability partner who helps motivate me to go to the gym and encourages me to eat healthy foods. Taking advantage of the challenges in JJ's private group only makes you stronger. It helps to keep your mind focused, giving you an understanding of what your body needs to be successful on this journey.

Remember that only you can make the choice to better

yourself. Believe that you can do it because this journey is all about your mind making the right decisions. There will be times when you have to replace people in your circle to find those who really support you. This is YOUR journey and only YOU can make goals to get YOU to where YOU want to be.

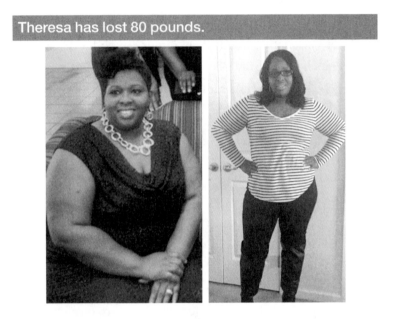

Theresa has lost 80 pounds.

My name is Theresa, and I have been on the Green Smoothie Cleanse journey for two years. I have lost 80 pounds and I'm down from a size 22/24 to a size 14 because of this new lifestyle!

I have known for years that I needed change and tried every fad "diet" out there. It was two years ago, on my birthday, that I made up my mind to do the Green Smoothie Cleanse. I'd taken a picture outside of my new house with my husband and kid and when I viewed the pictures I didn't look real. My face looked as if it had been blown up like a balloon. I was horrified.

I joined the Green Smoothie Cleanse Facebook group a couple months prior, but only looked around wondering if I could *really* do the program. However, once I saw the pictures of myself I made up my mind to start the 10-Day Green Smoothie Cleanse. I was both excited and determined. After five days, I'd lost 6 pounds and by day 10 I'd dropped an unbelievable 17 pounds! It was the beginning of my new lifestyle.

I don't have any more problems with anemia or low iron after following the Green Smoothie Cleanse and the Detox/ Hormonal Balance/Eat Clean/Mental Mastery/Move system. My acid reflux has disappeared, my blood pressure has improved tremendously, there are no more dizzy spells, and my joints do not ache. I can climb stairs, exercise, walk, and even run a little without feeling as though I am going to pass out! I feel amazing and everyone else even noticed that my skin is clear and more even-toned.

My motivation comes from my children, my husband, and my friends and family. In both the Green Smoothie Cleanse Facebook page and the VIP group, I notice others struggling and use what I've learned to motivate them. I am at a place where I feel as though I cannot fail. I have too many people counting on me and that is what keeps me going, along with prayer.

For anyone who needs encouragement on their journey, I say, stay the course! If you fall off, get right back on and keep moving towards your destination, whether it's weight loss or getting healthier overall. You owe it to yourself.

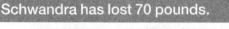

Schwandra has lost 70 pounds.

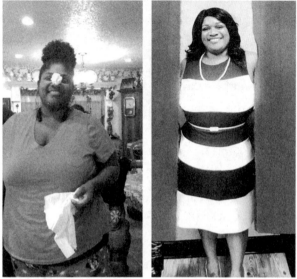

It was time to be a heathier me so that I could be around for my four blessings. My children absolutely deserve the best version of their mother. I began to search for diets that would work and was unsuccessful until I stumbled across JJ Smith's Green Smoothie Cleanse Facebook page. I stalked the page for two months and finally decided to order the *10-Day Green Smoothie Cleanse* book. I was still skeptical after receiving the book in the mail, and therefore waited another four months before actually purchasing the ingredients for the 10-day cleanse. By day 4, I was so amazed by how much energy I had, how much healthier my skin appeared, and how my shirts were beginning to fit me differently. I thought I was dreaming when I stepped on the scale on day 11—I'd lost 25 pounds! I began telling everyone how the Green Smoothie Cleanse changed my life.

I was at my highest weight when I started the Green

Smoothie Cleanse for the first time. I have now completed three 10-day cleanses in the past year. When I am not on the full 10-day cleanse, I stick to the modified version by enjoying a smoothie for breakfast, a healthy lunch, a smoothie for dinner, and healthy snacks in between my meals. When I began my journey, I was wearing a pant size 24/26, dress size 26, and shirt size 3X/4X. Ten months later, my pant size is 18, dress size 16, and shirt size XL. I have lost a total of 70 pounds!

The 10-Day Green Smoothie Cleanse has changed my life for the better. I have more energy to play with my children and my skin is glowing all of the time! The cleanse has also tremendously helped lower my blood pressure. My blood pressure is at an all-time low, and my doctor is so amazed by my health transformation.

I never want to be that unhealthy person sitting in my doctor's office again and that keeps me motivated. I want to be free and live a normal healthy life! JJ Smith's Facebook page has been one of my biggest motivations as well. You push yourself to keep going once you realize that you are not alone and you have wonderful people from all around the world supporting you. Not only do you want to do this for yourself, but along the way you are hoping your struggles and success will inspire others to keep thriving and going!

I know that every day I am getting healthier and healthier, and that strengthens my motivation. I want to be around to raise my kids and grandkids—when that day comes! I keep a positive mind-set at all times. I am grateful that I have found a realistic program that actually works. I am still able to enjoy good, yummy, healthy food! The one thing that I would say to encourage you on your journey is that you matter and to take it one day at a time. It did not take one day for you to gain the weight, and it is not going to take one day to get it all off. It is a process, just stay the course!

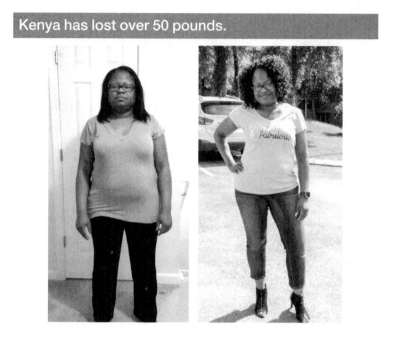

Kenya has lost over 50 pounds.

I heard about JJ Smith and the 10-Day Green Smoothie Cleanse long before I started on my journey to a healthier life-style. One of my former coworkers started the cleanse and I remember asking her, "How in the world do you *just* drink smoothies all day, because I would need to chew something?" She laughed and responded, "It isn't as bad as you think." She was right! I purchased JJ's book *10-Day Green Smoothie Cleanse* out of curiosity and started following the public group on Facebook. It was not until several months later that I joined "the movement."

I remember that day, that exact moment. I was at my favorite retail store trying on several pairs of pants for work. I needed new clothes because I'd gained even more weight, tipping the scales at 215 pounds. Nothing worked, nothing fit, and I was disgusted with myself for having gained so much weight over the past several years. My daughter, who was nine at the time, witnessed my moment of self-disgust. She sat in silence as I fussed at myself, watched me put everything back on the rack, and finally asked, "Mom, why are you putting everything back?" I told her that I was ready to lose weight, even after saying it repeatedly for so long—I was *really* ready. I walked out of the store, drove home, and sulked that evening. However, by the next morning everything changed.

What I failed to mention earlier is that I had recently joined a local fitness facility but never actually went to workout. I'd given myself a ton of excuses: I was not motivated, did not have time, and didn't know how to work the machines. I decided that the excuses had run out and if I was going to make a change I needed to take the first step. The answer to not having enough time was to make time. I'd just taken a voluntary leave from the workforce and suddenly possessed all of the time I needed to get started. I decided that while I was home, I would make good use of the time and focus on getting healthy. I picked up JJ's book that I purchased months earlier and next called the fitness facility to inquire about meeting with a trainer.

A year and a half ago my life changed forever. I started my very first cleanse and lost 7 pounds! Later that same week, I began working with a trainer. Since then, I have incorporated 10-day cleanses and exercise (two to three times per week) into my everyday life. I was able to wear many of the pants I had outgrown within my first four weeks. I went shopping again—in my closet!

I decided that I needed to have a physical after completing a couple of cleanses and meeting regularly with a trainer. I had not had a physical or any type of blood work done for almost ten years, but I knew that my cholesterol was high. I found a new doctor, made an appointment, and during my follow-up visit to discuss my blood work, she confirmed that my cholesterol was indeed high. By the time I actually saw the doctor, I had lost 26 pounds. After I informed her of by weight loss, she told me that without the weight loss my cholesterol would have been much higher. She was also very much interested in what I was doing to lose the weight and I began to share everything I knew about JJ Smith and the 10-Day Green Smoothie Cleanse.

My cholesterol is almost back to normal ranges and continues to improve each time I visit my doctor. I am very happy to say that I have lost 54 pounds and refuse to find that weight again! I have also lost 29¼ inches and over 16 percent of my body fat.

There are moments when I am weak and crave a soda or fried foods, but I stay motivated by knowing that I will be able to get into a pair of jeans or a sexy dress that I've seen in the store. I am also inspired by the nonscale victories and others' response to my success on this lifelong journey. I cannot tell other people about the strategies I use to maintain a healthy lifestyle and not live by them. It is all about the mental mastery JJ teaches!

My mind-set is simple: I will not go back to that place where I was not at my best! I was not at my best physically, mentally, or emotionally and I refuse to go back. The one thing that I would say to encourage you is to simply get started. Once you begin to see results, you will keep going.

**Linnell is a proud size 8.**

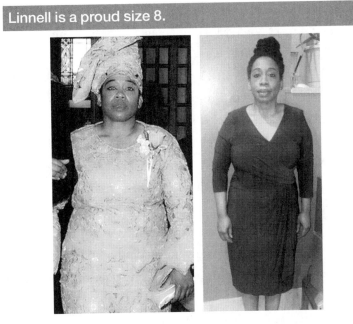

My journey towards health and wellness began with my annual visit to the doctor's office every November. I weighed in at a whopping 200 pounds and my blood pressure was 160/100. My doctor informed me that if my weight and blood pressure did not change, I would be taking additional medication.

It was nearing the holidays, one of the hardest times to change our diets and when Thanksgiving arrived I cooked, ate, and almost had a heart attack. Christmas then came which is also my daughter's birthday. I cooked our traditional feast and baked desserts, but this time around I made a vegetarian meal for myself. My family was visiting from Maryland during the holiday and my daughter prepared a vegetable and fruit smoothie for breakfast. I explained to her that these foods should never be mixed. My daughter then handed me some information to read about the smoothies she was blending. I requested to taste this green smoothie and the rest is history. When my daughter left for Maryland, I went home with her. I could hardly walk and was on steroids, Albuterol, Singulair, and Z-Pak.

I decided to do the 10-Day Green Smoothie Cleanse and I lost 10 pounds! After this, I joined the VIP support group and purchased my online books. It was not easy, but I was determined to change my health condition before I suffered a heart attack. Months earlier, I was so embarrassed by my weight that I'd stopped looking at myself in the mirror but now I was inspired to keep going.

I believe God gave me a second chance with JJ Smith's system. In February, I received my hormone therapy and my middle began to shrivel. My disposition also changed; I was both calmer and happier. In January, l was a size 14 and lost 15 pounds, come February I lost another 10 pounds. Over the course of the next four months, I'd lose 30 more pounds. In July, I was at a size 10 and by September, I moved to a size 8 while dropping an additional 5 pounds for a total weight loss of 60 pounds.

While detoxing my liver, I was also detoxing my brain as the two are connected. When you change your thoughts, you change your destiny.

# Appendix:

# Eat Clean and Balanced Foods to Achieve Healthy Weight Loss

---

## WHAT ARE CLEAN AND BALANCED FOODS?

Clean foods are primarily natural, whole, raw, or organic—foods that the body can effectively digest and utilize for energy without leaving excess waste or toxins in the body. Clean foods include lean proteins, good carbs, and healthy fats. Balanced foods mean that you will balance your meals by eating protein every time you eat a carbohydrate. So, if you have carbohydrates, you want to always include protein. Maintaining this balance between proteins and carbs is a very simple but incredibly effective method for preventing insulin spikes and aiding the body in burning fat.

Why protein every time you eat? Protein counteracts the body's overreaction to carbohydrates, which cause insulin spikes and fat storage. Proteins will also help you feel full longer and thus will help prevent overeating and food cravings. Protein will also help you build and maintain muscle mass and, as we've learned, muscle naturally burns more calories than fat.

Eating clean and balanced foods will help you lose weight for all of the following reasons:

- It will help you address the underlying reasons your body stores fat.
- You will learn which foods will help you stay thin and maintain your healthy weight.
- You will have more control over your insulin and blood sugar levels.
- You will burn fat, especially the belly fat and love handles.
- You will gain control of your appetite and cravings.

## TWELVE PRINCIPLES FOR CLEAN AND BALANCED EATING

To complement the strategies in this book, you can follow these twelve guiding principles for eating clean and balanced foods to help you achieve your weight-loss goals. Look at the principles below as your instructions on how to eat clean and balanced foods.

- **PRINCIPLE #1:** Choose nutrient-rich foods, not empty calories. This means you will eat foods that are high in vitamins, minerals, phytonutrients, fiber, and omega-3 fatty acids. Eating junk foods is like eating empty calories. You want your calories to provide you with nutritional benefits that will help you heal your body and maintain a permanently healthy weight. Before you eat anything, ask yourself, is this a healthy, nutrient-rich food or empty calories? Commit to be mindful of everything you eat.

- **PRINCIPLE #2:** Eat protein with every meal, and eat it first before the carbohydrates or fats. You can also eat protein by itself. Eating protein foods does not cause insulin spikes, making them an important staple of eating clean and balanced foods.

- **PRINCIPLE #3:** Always "balance" carbohydrates with protein. Whenever you eat a carbohydrate, eat some protein along with it. As a general guideline, the protein should be about half the amount of the carbohydrates. For example, if you had 30 grams of carbohydrates, then eat about 15 grams of protein along with it to prevent insulin spikes that cause excess fat to be stored in the body. You can use food labels to determine how much carbs (or "net carbs") and protein is in food. (See the examples at the end of this section to better understand how to balance carbohydrates with protein at each meal.)

- **PRINCIPLE #4:** Don't overeat carbohydrates. It is important to not overeat carbohydrates. Limit yourself to no more than two servings of high-carbohydrate foods at any one meal or snack. This will prevent excess carbohydrates from being stored as fat. If you are still hungry, then eat more vegetables to satisfy your hunger. Do not try to eat other high-carbohydrate foods, which will convert to fat in your body, or too much protein, which will hinder weight loss by adding extra calories. One serving of high-carbohydrate foods is about ½ cup or 15 grams of carbohydrates. So, the maximum amount of high-carb foods you should eat at any one meal is two servings, which is 30 grams or about 1 cup, always balanced with a high-protein food.

- **PRINCIPLE #5:** Avoid excessive sugar, salt, and trans fat. We discussed a number of foods that cause weight gain and are bad for your health. However, these three are at the top of the list. Try to avoid them at all costs. They have no nutritional value and are simply bad for your health. If you are interested in learning more, chapter 3 in my book *Lose Weight Without Dieting or Working Out* is entirely devoted to explaining how detrimental sugar is. Salt is also bad for your health and causes bloating, swelling, and fluid retention. As far as trans fat, the good news is that the FDA regulates it, and food manufacturers now have to list how much trans fat is in each serving when trans fats exceeds 0.5 grams per serving.

- **PRINCIPLE #6:** Eat at least five servings of fruits and veggies each day. Fruit breaks down faster in the body than any other food, leaving us fueled and energized, and because it is a highly cleansing food, it leaves no toxic residue and acts as a strong cleanser for the body. You need to eat vegetables if you want to get thin, as studies have shown that those who eat a large variety of vegetables have the least amount of body fat. Veggies and fruits are naturally balanced because they contain both protein and carbohydrates. They are made up of mostly water and fiber, so they can be eaten in larger quantities. However, there are a few exceptions. Consumption of corn and potatoes should be minimal and, of course, always be balanced with protein. Green smoothies are also a great way to get lots of fruits and veggies into your diet.

- **PRINCIPLE #7:** Limit your intake of red meat to two to three times per week. Red meat contains a lot of saturated fat, so try to limit your intake to two or three times a week. Instead, eat more protein from fish, poultry, and vegetable sources, such as brown rice, beans, and nuts, which contain good essential fats.

- **PRINCIPLE #8:** Eat two healthy snacks per day. Snacks keep you from getting hungry between meals. Eating snacks allows you to feed your body every three to four hours, which keeps your metabolism revved up. See the list of healthy snacks provided later in this chapter.

- **PRINCIPLE #9:** Eat at least 30 grams of fiber per day. Numerous studies have shown that high-fiber diets help you lose weight and protect against heart disease, stroke, and certain kinds of cancer. Chapter 8 in *Lose Weight Without Dieting or Working Out* provides a list of foods that are high in fiber as well as fiber supplements that help you to eat 30 grams of fiber per day.

- **PRINCIPLE #10:** Drink Plenty of Water Daily. It's important to drink plenty of water and stay hydrated. Drinking water helps boost your metabolism, cleanse your body of waste and toxins, and decrease your appetite. Additionally, drinking more water will help you reduce fluid retention and release water weight. The goal would be to drink half your body weight in ounces. So, as an example, if you weigh 220 pounds, that would be drinking 110 ounces of water per day.

- **PRINCIPLE #11:** Eat four to five times a day. You will lose weight more quickly if you eat four or five times a day as opposed to only three meals (or fewer). Try to eat every three to four hours, and think in terms of three meals and two healthy snacks. Each time you eat, you stimulate your metabolism for a short period of time; thus, the more often you eat, the more you speed up your metabolism. Eating every two to three hours feeds your muscles and starves fat.

- **PRINCIPLE #12:** Buy organic as much as possible. Buy organic foods, which don't have chemical preservatives, food additives, hormones, pesticides, and antibiotics. Fresh, organic foods are far less toxic than highly processed and packaged/frozen foods and leave less residue and waste in the body.

## "CLEAN AND BALANCED" FOOD CHOICES

You can eat clean and balanced foods from the lean proteins, good carbs, and healthy fats lists below. This section provides specific lists of some food choices for each category. This list is meant to give you many food choice options, but it does not represent the only foods that are suitable for healthy weight loss. Always use the principles above to select the right balance of lean proteins, good carbs, and healthy fats each day. The result will provide the best balance of carbs, proteins, and fats to ensure that the rate at which your body breaks down your food into energy lends itself to meeting your weight-loss goals.

The following are daily guidelines for how much of each type of food to eat for a well-balanced diet.

- *Lean proteins* (30 percent of daily diet): 2 or 3 servings (3 to 4 ounces per serving) of lean proteins, such as lean red meat, poultry, and fish
- *Good carbs* (45 percent of daily diet): At least 5 servings of fruits and vegetables/legumes (beans) and 2 or 3 servings of whole grains (½ cup = one serving)
- *Healthy fats* (25 percent of daily diet): 1 to 2 servings (about 1 ounce) of nuts and seeds per day and 1 to 3 tablespoons of healthy oils

# Lean Proteins

*Eat 2 or 3 servings (3 to 4 ounces per serving) of lean protein daily.*

| Fish and Shellfish | Chicken and Turkey | Lean Red Meat | Dairy Products |
|---|---|---|---|
| bass, calamari, catfish, clams, cod, crabmeat, flounder, grouper, haddock, halibut, lobster, mackerel, oysters, perch, wild salmon, sardines, scallops, shrimp, red snapper, sole, tilapia, trout, tuna | skinless chicken breasts, skinless Cornish hen, skinless turkey breast | lean beef, flank steak, sirloin, top round, London broil, pork tenderloin, pork rib chops, pork roast | protein drink/ powder, goat and sheep's milk products, unsweetened yogurt, nondairy milk such as unsweetened almond, rice, hemp, soy milk |

# Good Carbs

*Fruits: 2 servings or 2 whole fruits daily*

*Veggies/legumes: 3 to 4 cups daily*

*Whole grains: 2 to 3 three servings daily (½ cup = one serving)*

| Fruits | Veggies/Legumes | Whole Grains |
|---|---|---|
| apples, apricots, avocado, bananas, blackberries, blueberries, cantaloupe, cherries, cranberries, dates, figs, grapes, grapefruit, guava, honeydew, kiwi, lemon, lime, mango, nectarines, oranges, papaya, peaches, pears, pineapple, plums, pomegranate, prunes, raspberries, strawberries, tangerines, watermelon | alfalfa, artichokes, asparagus, beets and beet greens, broccoli, Brussels sprouts, cabbage, carrots, cauliflower, celery, chilies, cilantro, collard greens, cucumbers, dandelion greens, eggplant, fennel, garlic, green beans, kale, kelp, leeks, lettuce, mushrooms, mustard greens, okra, onion, parsley, parsnips, pea pods, peas, peppers, pumpkin, radishes, rhubarb, rutabaga, scallions, spinach, summer squash, sweet potato, tomato, turnips, turnip greens, watercress, yams, zucchini, black beans, lentils, kidney beans, pinto beans, split peas, chickpeas (garbanzo beans), lima beans, butter beans, wax beans | barley, bran, brown rice, buckwheat, bulgur wheat, cornmeal, millet, oat bran, oatmeal, oats, quinoa, rye spelt, wheat germ, wild rice, whole grain/gluten-free breads, whole grain/gluten-free pastas, whole grain cereals |

# Healthy Fats

*Nuts and Seeds: 2 or 3 servings (about 1 ounce) of nuts and seeds daily*

*Healthy oils: 1 to 3 tablespoons daily*

| Nuts | Seeds | Healthy Oils |
|------|-------|--------------|
| almonds, Brazil nuts, cashews, coconut, hazelnuts, macadamia nuts, pistachios, pecans, walnuts | ground flaxseeds, pumpkin seeds, sesame seeds, sunflower seeds | avocado oil, canola oil, coconut oil, extra-virgin olive oil, flaxseed oil, fish oil, sesame oil, walnut oil |

# Healthy Snacks

*Eat 2 healthy snacks per day.*

| Healthy Low-Calorie Fruits and Veggies (Less than 100 calories) | Healthy Low-Calorie Nuts and Seeds (Raw or Dry Roasted) (Less than 100 Calories) | Healthy High-Protein/ Low-Fat Snacks |
|---|---|---|
| 1 large apple | 12 raw almonds | 1 hard-boiled egg |
| ½ cup of unsweetened applesauce | 8 walnut halves | 2 oz. tuna, lightly salted |
| 1 medium grapefruit | 4 Brazil nuts | ½ cup low-fat cottage cheese |
| 1 medium pear | 3/4 oz. pumpkin seeds | 1 oz. string goat cheese |
| 1 medium banana | 2 tablespoons sunflower seeds | 1 cup plain fat-free yogurt |
| 1 cup blueberries | 20 macadamia nuts | 8 baked tortilla chips with 3 tablespoons salsa |
| 1 cup blackberries | 20 peanuts | 5 cups plain popcorn |
| 1 cup of raspberries | | |
| 1 cup of fresh cherries | | |
| 1 large nectarine | | |
| 2 medium peaches | | |
| 2 cups of grapes | | |
| 2 kiwis | | |
| 1 cup of celery/celery sticks | | |
| ½ cup of baby carrots | | |
| 1 cup of broccoli | | |
| 1 cup of cauliflower | | |

# Conclusion

Over the years, I've witnessed the power individuals have to change virtually anything and everything in their lives in an instant. Everything we need to turn our dreams into a reality is within us. We are fully equipped to achieve our weight-loss goals.

No more looking for excuses for why you're overweight. Something deep down inside of you is telling you it's time to change. The fact that you're reading this book is evidence that you are the type of person who can change. There is a greater force at work telling you that you can benefit from the information within the pages of this book. You will not only have the body you desire, but you will live your very best life.

Can you imagine a life where you look in the mirror and love what you see? Can you imagine having vibrant energy to enjoy time with your family and friends? Can you imagine a life where you are in control of your health and your weight and no longer struggle with thoughts of emotional eating? All of these things are waiting for you. It is time to upgrade your life. If you still haven't gotten to your goal weight, it's time to try something different because you deserve it.

I hope this book has challenged you to use the God-given power within you to transform your mind, body, and spirit. I've provided tips and strategies that will allow you to produce measurable, long-lasting changes to achieve your health and weight-loss goals. No matter how well you've done sticking to your diet or weight-loss plan, you want more. You want to experience a life full of accomplishments with your body, career, and personal relationships. You want to experience a life much greater than the one you live. Deep down inside, you know you are destined for greatness, whether it's as a mother, father, professional, or friend. I know this because you bought this book and have read it. Most people buy a book and never read it, but you've read through to the end. You have taken the first step to producing amazing results in your life.

In closing, I want to leave you with my *Ten Commandments for Looking Young and Feeling Great,* which I always share at the end of my teleseminars and speeches.

1. *Thou shalt love thyself.* Self-love is essential to survival. There is no successful, authentic relationship with others without self-love. We cannot water the land from a dry well. Self-love is not selfish or self-indulgent. We have to take care of our needs first so we can give to others from abundance.

2. *Thou shalt take responsibility for thine own health and well-being.* If you want to be healthy, have more energy, and feel great, you must take the time to learn what is involved and apply it to your own life. You have to watch what goes into your mouth, how much exercise and physical activity you get, and what thoughts you're thinking throughout the day.

3. *Thou shalt sleep.* Sleep and rest is the body's way of re-charging the system. Sleep is the easiest yet most un-derrated activity for healing the body. Lack of sleep definitely saps your glow and instantly ages you, giving you puffy red eyes with dark circles under them.

4. *Thou shalt detoxify and cleanse the body.* Detoxifying the body means ridding the body of poisons and toxins so that you can speed up weight loss and restore great health. A clean body is a beautiful body!

5. *Thou shalt remember that a healthy body is a sexy body.* Real women's bodies look beautiful! It's about getting healthy and having style and confidence and wearing clothes that match your body type.

6. *Thou shalt eat healthy, natural, whole foods.* Healthy eat-ing can turn back the hands of time and return the body to a more youthful state. When you eat natural foods, you simply look and feel better. You keep the body clean at the cellular level and look radiant despite your age. Eating healthy should be part of your "beauty regimen."

7. *Thou shalt embrace healthy aging.* The goal is not to stop the aging process but to embrace it. Healthy aging is staying healthy as you age, which is looking and feel-ing great despite your age.

8. *Thou shalt commit to a lifestyle change.* Losing weight permanently requires a commitment to change: in your thinking, your lifestyle, your mind-set. It requires gaining knowledge and making permanent changes in your life for the better!

9. *Thou shalt embrace the journey.* This is a journey that will change your life. It's not a diet, it's a lifestyle! Be

kind and supportive to yourself. Learn to applaud yourself for the smallest accomplishment. And when you slip up sometimes, know that it is okay—it is called being human.

10. *Thou shalt live, love, and laugh.* Laughter is good for the soul. Live your life with passion! Never give up on your dreams! And most importantly—love! Remember that love never fails!

Now that you have a new perspective on weight loss, be sure to share your experience with others and help them produce measurable, long-lasting changes to achieve their health and weight-loss goals.

# About the Author

www.JJSmithOnline.com

JJ Smith is a #1 *New York Times* bestselling author, nutritionist and certified weight-loss expert, passionate relationship/life coach, and inspirational speaker. She has been featured on *The Dr. Oz Show*, *The Steve Harvey Show*, *The View*, *The Montel Williams Show*, *The Jamie Foxx Show*, and *The Michael Baisden Show*. JJ has made appearances on the NBC, FOX, CBS, CNN, and CW Network television stations, as well as in the pages of *Glamour*, *Essence*, *Heart and Soul*, and *Ladies Home Journal*. Since reclaiming her health, losing weight, and discovering a "second youth" in her forties, bestselling author JJ Smith has become the voice of inspiration to those who want to lose weight, be healthy, and get their sexy back. JJ Smith provides lifestyle solutions for losing weight, getting healthy, looking younger, and improving your love life.

JJ has dedicated her life to the field of healthy eating and living. JJ's passion is to educate others and share with them the natural remedies to stay slim, restore health, and look and feel younger. JJ has studied many philosophies of natural healing and learned from some of the great teachers of our time. After studying and applying knowledge about how to heal the body and lose weight, JJ received several certifications; she is a certified nutritionist and a certified weight-management expert. JJ received certification as a Weight-Management Specialist from the National Exercise and Sports Trainers Association (NESTA). She is also a member of the American Nutrition Association (ANA).

JJ's current *New York Times* bestseller, *Green Smoothies for Life*, provides a 30-Day Program that teaches you how to lose 20 pounds in thirty days by incorporating green smoothies, healthy meals, and desserts into their eating regimen and discover an approach to eating for the rest of your life. JJ's previous book, a #1 *New York Times* bestseller, *the 10-Day Green Smoothie Cleanse,* is a proven plan to safely and quickly detoxify the body, and jump-start weight loss. Most people who follow the plan strictly experience weight loss of up to 15 pounds in only ten days.

JJ holds a BA in mathematics from Hampton University in Virginia. She continued her education at the The Wharton Business School in the Executive Management Certificate program. She currently serves as vice president and partner of the IT consulting firm, Intact Technology, Inc., in Greenbelt, Maryland. JJ was also the youngest African American to receive a vice president position at a Fortune 500 company. Her hobbies include reading, writing, and deejaying.

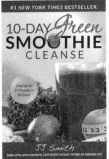
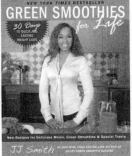
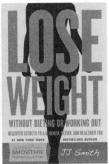

"Delight thine self also in the Lord. And he shall give you the desires of thine heart.

Psalms 37:4.